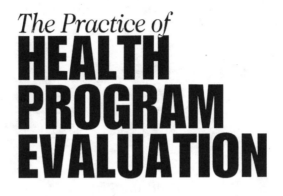

The Practice of
HEALTH PROGRAM EVALUATION

To Aunt Imogene

Acknowledgments

In many ways, this book is a synthesis of what I have learned about evaluation from my evaluation teachers and colleagues, and I am very grateful for what they have given me. I wish to acknowledge and thank my teachers—Marilyn Bergner and Stephen Shortell—who provided the bedrock for my professional career in health program evaluation when I was in graduate school. In those days, their program evaluation class was structured around a new, unpublished book, *Health Program Evaluation*, by Stephen Shortell and William Richardson, which has since become a classic in our field and provided a model for this work. I also thank Donald Miller, my urban planning professor, for his insights and cutting-edge methods of conducting plan evaluation. I give my special thanks to Ann Blalock, who introduced me to the politics of programs in the real world and who was a role model for navigating this terrain with grace and humor.

As a new professor and beginning teacher, I benefited greatly from the support and help of other teachers of health program evaluation. I wish to thank Ronald Andersen, who taught health program evaluation at the University of Chicago (now at UCLA) for many years. He was an early role model and shared many insights about how to package course material in ways that could be grasped readily by graduate students. His evaluation course divided the evaluation process into three distinct phases, and I discovered early that his model also worked very well in my own evaluation courses. I also wish to thank Diane

Martin and Rita Altamore, who taught this course at the University of Washington and shared their approaches in teaching this subject with me. I especially want to thank the speakers in my evaluation course for their insights about the practice of program evaluation: Tom Wickizer (design and conduct of program evaluation), Sharyne Shiu-Thornton (conducting evaluation in a cultural context), Beti Thompson (community-based program evaluation), Cynthia Curreri (use of evaluation results in decision making), and Dan Lessler and Nicole Urban (cost-effectiveness analysis). I also benefited greatly from "lessons learned" about evaluation through my work with other faculty—Michael Chapko, Douglas Conrad, Paula Diehr, Mary Durham, Louis Fiset, Peter Milgrom, Donald Patrick, and others at the University of Washington, as well as Don Dillman and John Tarnai at Washington State University.

Several people played important roles in the production of this book. I wish to thank the W. K. Kellogg Foundation for its generous grant award, which created the time and opportunity for me to write this book. I also wish to thank everyone who provided comments on previous versions of this book. I especially want to thank the students in my health program evaluation class, particularly Letitia Reason and Henry Espinoza, for providing detailed comments for each chapter. Many thanks also are extended to the Sage reviewers. Their thoughtful comments significantly improved the quality of this textbook: Ronald Andersen, University of California, Los Angeles; Robin Lin Miller, University of Illinois at Chicago; William L. Miller, MD, Lehigh Valley Hospital, Allentown, Pennsylvania; Lynn Overman, University of Alabama at Birmingham; and Letitia Reason, University of Washington.

I am extremely grateful for the patience and help that I received from my secretary, Alice Gronski, in producing the final manuscript. Her organizational skills and attention to detail were invaluable in completing the final manuscript. I also thank and acknowledge the efforts of Laura Hammond and Daniel Moore, who provided administrative support for producing earlier versions of the textbook.

Finally, I thank my family, as well as my mother and father, and siblings Linda and Gary—for their patience, support, and encouragement in this effort.

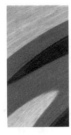

PROLOGUE

CHAPTER 1

Health Program Evaluation

Is It Worth It?

Evaluation is a part of everyday life. Does Ford make a better truck than Chevrolet? What are the reviews of the new movie? What are the top 10 football teams in the country? Who will be the recipient of this year's outstanding teacher award? All these questions entail judgments of worth reached by weighing information against some explicit or implicit yardstick (Weiss 1972). When judgments result in decisions, evaluation is being performed at some level (Shortell and Richardson 1978).

This book is about the evaluation of health programs and the role it plays in program management and decision making. All societies face sundry health problems. Accidents, cancer, diabetes, heart disease, HIV infection, inequitable access to health care, influenza, suicide, and others are mentioned commonly in the health literature (McGinnis and Foege 1993). A *health program* is an organized response to reduce or eliminate one or more problems by achieving one or more objectives, with the ultimate goal of improving the health of society (Shortell and Richardson 1978).

The purpose of *evaluation* is to produce information about the performance of a program in achieving its objectives. In general, most evaluations are conducted to answer two fundamental questions: Is the program working as intended? and Why is this the case? Research methods are applied to answer these questions and to increase the accuracy and objectivity of judgments about the program's success in reaching its objectives. The evaluation process fulfills this purpose by defining clear and explicit criteria for success, collecting representative evidence of program performance, and comparing it to the criteria established at the outset. Evaluations help program managers understand the reasons for program performance, which may lead to improvement or refinement of the program. Evaluations also help program funders to make informed judgments about a program's worth, which may result in decisions to extend it to other sites or to cut back or abolish a program so that resources may be allocated elsewhere. In essence, evaluation is a management or decision-making tool for program administrators, planners, policymakers, and other health officials.

From a societal perspective, evaluation also may be viewed as a deliberate means of promoting social change for the betterment of society (Shortell and Richardson 1978; Weiss 1972). Just as personal growth and development are fundamental to a person's quality of life, so do organizations and institutions mature by learning more about their own behavior (Shortell and Richardson 1978). The value of evaluation comes from the insights that its findings can generate, which can speed up the learning process to produce benefits on a societal scale (Cronbach 1987).

Evaluation, however, can be a double-edged sword. The desire to learn more is often accompanied by the fear of what may be found (Shortell and Richardson 1978). On the one hand, favorable results typically are greeted with a sigh of relief by those who want the program to succeed. On the other hand, unfavorable results may be as welcome as the plague. When an evaluation finds that a program has not achieved its objectives, the very worth of the program is often brought into question. Program managers and staff may feel threatened by poor evaluation results because they often are held accountable for them by funders, who may decide the program has little worth. In this case, funders or other decision makers often have the power and authority to change program implementation, replace personnel, or even terminate the program and allocate funds elsewhere.

For popular health programs, such as prenatal care for low-income women, program advocates may view unfavorable results as a threat to the very life of the program. To a great degree, the worth of prenatal care programs is grounded on the argument that public spending now will prevent future costs and medical complications associated with low birth weight (Huntington and Connell 1994). Previous evaluations reported "good" news: Prenatal care pays for itself (for every $1.00 spent, up to $3.38 will be saved). The "bad" news is that the evaluations have serious methodological flaws that may have resulted in overestimates of the cost savings from prenatal care (Huntington and Connell 1994). These findings have attracted national attention because they challenge the very worth of prenatal care programs *if* the objective of those programs is to save more than they cost (Kolata 1994).

In all evaluations, the worth of a program depends on both its performance and the desirability of its objectives, which is always a question of values (Kane et al. 1974; Palumbo 1987; Weiss 1983). For prenatal care and other prevention programs, the real question may not be "How much does this save?" but more simply, "How much is this program worth?" (Huntington and Connell 1994). For health and all types of social programs, the answer to this fundamental question can have far-reaching consequences for large numbers of people.

GROWTH OF HEALTH PROGRAM EVALUATION

Evaluation is a relatively new discipline. Prior to the 1960s, formal evaluations of social and health programs were conducted rarely, and few professionals performed evaluations as a full-time career (Shadish et al. 1991). With the election of Lyndon Johnson to the presidency in 1964, the United States entered into an era of unprecedented growth in social and health programs for the disadvantaged. Medicare, Medicaid, and other health care programs were launched, and Congress often mandated and funded evaluation of their performance (Anderson 1985). As public and private funding for evaluation grew, so did the number of professionals and agencies conducting evaluations. Today, evaluation is a well-known, international profession. In many countries, evaluators have established professional associations (e.g., the American Evaluation Association and the Canadian Evaluation Society) that hold annual conferences. Although an association for health program evaluation does not exist in the United States, the Association for Health Services Research, the American Public Health Association, and other groups often serve as national forums for health evaluators to collaborate and disseminate their findings.

Other forces also have contributed to the growth of health program evaluation over the past three decades. Two important factors are the *escalating costs* of health services and *managed care*. Between 1989 and 1996, the nation's health bill grew from $604 billion to more than $1 trillion, with the public share increasing from 40% to 47% (Levit et al. 1997; Levit et al. 1991). Faced with higher costs, employers, government, and other purchasers have abandoned traditional fee-for-service (FFS) medical coverage and are contracting with a variety of managed care organizations (MCOs), which deliver health services through networks of participating physicians and hospitals (Grembowski et al. 1998). To control costs in their networks, MCOs impose a variety of constraints and incentives on physician behavior through utilization review, financial incentives, and other management systems. As more and more Americans obtain their health care through MCOs, it becomes more important to understand how MCOs control utilization and whether the utilization controls they impose affect access and service delivery, health outcomes, and satisfaction (Grembowski et al. 1998; Schlesinger 1986; Sisk et al. 1996; Udvarhelyi et al. 1991). Evaluation is a tool for examining the influence of managed care on the performance of health care systems.

The large expenditures, in turn, have increased the importance of *accountability* for the public and private dollars invested in health programs and medical services (Shadish et al. 1991; Shortell and McNerney 1990; Shortell and Richardson 1978). For financial and legal reasons, Congress and other funding agencies are concerned with holding programs accountable for funds and their disbursement, with an eye toward avoiding inappropriate payments. For performance reasons, funding agencies also want to know if their investments actually produced expected benefits while avoiding harmful side effects. Similarly, employers, government, and other purchasers of health services are concerned with clinical and fiscal accountability, or evidence that health care systems and providers deliver services of demonstrated efficacy and quality in an efficient manner (Relman 1988). Employers also want to know whether their investments in health care improve the productivity of their employees, for example, by collecting information about how quickly workers are back on the job after an episode of care (Moskowitz 1998).

A related factor is *scarce resources* for health programs. All societies have limited resources to address pressing health problems. When resources are scarce, competition for funds can intensify, and decision makers may allocate resources only to programs that can demonstrate good performance. In such environments, evaluations can provide useful information for managing programs, and if performance is sound, for defending the program's worth and justifying continued funding. If, however, an evaluation is launched solely to collect information to defend the program's worth in political battles over resource allocation, and if the evaluation is conducted in an impartial manner, there is no guarantee that an evaluation will produce results favoring the program.

Another factor stimulating interest in program evaluation is more emphasis on *prevention*. Many people and health professionals believe that prevention is better than cure. Because the evidence indicates that much disease is preventable (U.S. Department of Health and Human Services [DHHS] 1991), a wide variety of preventive programs and technologies have emerged to maintain or improve the nation's health. For example, immunizations to prevent disease, water fluoridation to reduce caries, mammography screening to detect breast cancer, and campaigns promoting the use of bicycle helmets to prevent injuries are common in our society. *Healthy People 2000* and its successor, *Healthy People 2010*, specify health promotion and disease prevention objectives for the nation and provide a framework for the development and implementation of federal, state, and local programs to meet these objectives (U.S. DHHS 1991). As the number of programs has proliferated, so has interest in evaluating their performance in achieving their objectives.

The growth of managed care also has stimulated interest in prevention. When providers are paid a fixed amount of money for delivering health services to an enrolled population (a form of payment known as capitation), providers have financial incentives to keep people healthy. Many managed care organizations have developed their own health promotion programs or partnered with local health departments to achieve common prevention goals (Coile 1997; Schlesinger and Gray 1998). In all these contexts, evaluation is a useful tool for identifying the effectiveness of these programs and the conditions when they are most successful (Hulscher et al. 1999). As mentioned earlier, however, although prevention and the diagnosis and treatment of illness in its early stages are often advocated because they can save health dollars, there is little evidence to support this argument (Russell 1993).

Another trend encouraging evaluation is the movement toward *evidence-based medicine*. More than 50 years of research have confirmed repeatedly that the practice patterns of physicians vary widely for similar patients from one health care setting to another (Blumenthal 1994). The fact that physicians treat similar patients in widely different ways has raised questions about the knowledge base of medicine. The knowledge vacuum, in turn, has encouraged MCOs to challenge the medical decisions of physicians in an effort to control their costs of care. In response, outcomes research has blossomed to identify those processes of care associated with good outcomes, and to encourage physicians to follow them (Blumenthal 1994; Kane 1997). The trend toward evidence-based medicine and outcomes research also is promoting health program evaluation, because both seek to understand the association between process and outcomes.

Over the past three decades, health program evaluation also has been promoted by public agencies, foundations, and other groups, which have sponsored a wide variety of *demonstration projects* to improve the performance of the health care system. Health professionals are constantly searching for new ways to improve the performance of the health care system. Consistent with our nation's belief in incrementalism in political decision making (Marmor 1998; Shortell and Richardson 1978), decision makers often desire information about whether a proposed change will actually work before authorizing changes on a broad scale. To supply this information, decision makers may approve demonstration projects or large-scale social experiments to test the viability of promising solutions to pressing health problems. Examples of large-scale demonstrations include programs to increase access to health services for low-income groups in central cities (Fleming and Andersen 1986) and interventions to reduce infant mortality in rural areas by improving perinatal care (Gortmaker et al. 1987), but perhaps the most prominent example is the Rand Health Insurance Study (Newhouse 1991). In a large-scale experiment, households were randomly assigned to health insurance plans with different cost-sharing arrangements to determine their impacts on use, expenditures, health outcomes, and satisfaction with medical and dental care. Evaluation is an important element of these and other demonstration projects because it provides the evidence for judging their success. Because large-scale evaluations are relatively expensive to conduct, controversy may exist about whether their findings are worth the resources invested in them. Nevertheless, decision makers are likely to continue authorizing such programs because they often address critical issues in health policy and because they give decision makers the flexibility to be responsive to a problem while avoiding long-term commitments of resources.

A final force stimulating the growth in health program evaluation is the growth of *administration*. Between 1968 and 1993, management and related personnel in medical care grew 692%, and financial administrative support increased by 308% (Himmelstein et al. 1996). Administrative occupations accounted for 18% of all medical personnel in 1968 and 27% in 1993. In addition, as managed care has grown in recent years, the relative power of administrators in the health care system also has increased (Srinivasan et al. 1998). These trends are important for health program evaluation because administration is grounded in the rational model of decision making, where resource allocation and other decisions are based partly on evidence of organization performance. Because a key function of evaluation is to produce information about program implementation and outcomes, administrators are major consumers of evaluation information, which can be used to make informed decisions about the management of the program. The greater number and greater clout of administrators have likely generated more interest in the evaluation of key programs and the use of evaluation findings in administrative decisions.

As a whole, the forces contributing to the growth of health program evaluation are interrelated and will likely continue into the foreseeable future. From these trends, three broad types of health program evaluation have emerged. They are reviewed in the next section.

TYPES OF HEALTH PROGRAM EVALUATION

Health programs usually are implemented to achieve specific outcomes by performing some type of intervention or service. In general, three basic types of evaluation are conducted in the health field:

▶ The evaluation of health programs

▶ The evaluation of the health care system

▶ The evaluation of health services

Evaluation of Health Programs

This type of evaluation includes programs created to reduce or eliminate a health problem or achieve a specific objective. *Healthy People 2010*, the national effort to set health objectives for the next decade, has established 20 "focus areas" for improving the nation's health, ranging from impairment and disability to violent and abusive behavior (see Figure 1.1).

In essence, the focus areas are a comprehensive inventory of the categories of health programs that can be implemented to achieve specific health objectives. For example, water fluoridation programs are implemented to improve oral health (area 15), or exercise programs are created to increase physical activity (area 3). The first type of evaluation assesses the performance of programs developed to achieve health objectives in these and other areas.

Evaluation of the Health Care System

The second type of evaluation is designed to produce knowledge about the performance of the health care system. Aday and colleagues (1998) present a framework for conducting evaluations of system performance based partly on Donabedian's (1973) earlier work (see Figure 1.2). A health care system has a *structure* defined by federal, state, and local laws and regulations; the availability of personnel, facilities, and other resources; and the organization and financing of care. The structure component also includes the characteristics of the population that the system serves, as well as the physical, social, and economic environments where they live. As a whole, the structure of the system influences

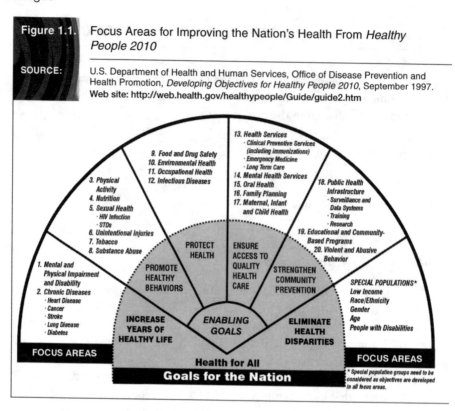

Figure 1.1. Focus Areas for Improving the Nation's Health From *Healthy People 2010*

SOURCE: U.S. Department of Health and Human Services, Office of Disease Prevention and Health Promotion, *Developing Objectives for Healthy People 2010*, September 1997. Web site: http://web.health.gov/healthypeople/Guide/guide2.htm

the *process* or delivery of health services, which in turn produces *outcomes,* both intermediate and ultimate. Intermediate outcomes are the three "Es" of system performance; they define what improvements in health and satisfaction (effectiveness) were produced by health services at what cost (efficiency) and for what population groups (equity). A fourth "E" (ethics) is essential for judging whether a fair or equitable distribution of the costs and outcomes of health services exists among those who deserve care and those who pay for it. Based on ethical principles of distributive justice, inequitable access to care exists when those who need care the most do not get it. Intermediate outcomes ultimately produce improvements in health and well-being, or quality of life.

Evaluations of system performance typically examine the influence of the structural component on the process of care, or the influence of the structure and process components on the outcomes of care (Clancy and Eisenberg 1998; Kane 1997). For example, an evaluation of the association between the structure and process components of the system was performed by Conrad and associates (1998), who examined whether patients' utilization of health services was

Figure 1.2.   Framework for Classifying Topics and Issues in Health Services Research

SOURCE: Reprinted with permission from *Evaluating the Healthcare System: Effectiveness, Efficiency, and Equity*, 2nd ed., by Lu Ann Aday, Charles Begley, David R. Lairson, and Carl Slater (Chicago: Health Administration Press, 1998), Figure 1.4.

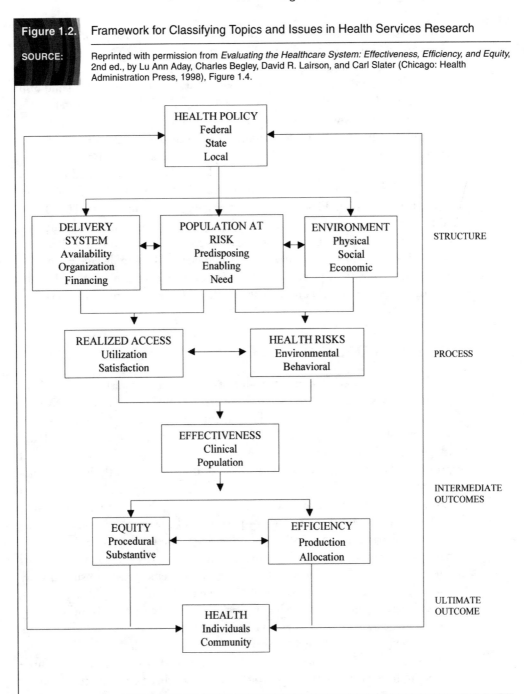

influenced by how the patients' primary care physicians were paid. The evaluation predicted that utilization would be greater among patients seeing primary care physicians paid fee-for-service than patients seeing physicians paid by salary. No association was detected, however, between payment method and utilization rates. Instead, higher patient age, female gender, richer plan benefits, and younger physicians were related to higher utilization rates.

Similarly, the Medical Outcomes Study performed an evaluation of the associations between the structure and outcomes of the system. In one of several publications from the study, Ware and colleagues (1996) addressed equity issues in system performance when they examined whether the type of health plan, fee-for-service (FFS) vs. health maintenance organization (HMO), affected health outcomes. They found that physical and mental health outcomes were similar for the average patient; however, patients who were elderly and poor with chronic illnesses were more than twice as likely to decline in physical health in HMOs than in FFS systems. No consistent pattern in mental health outcomes between HMO and FFS systems was detected for these patients.

Evaluation of Health Services

Whereas the second type of evaluation looks at the performance of the health care system, the third type of evaluation examines the cost-effectiveness of specific health services provided to patients in the system. The focus is measurement of the benefits, or health outcomes, of a medical technology relative to the costs of producing them. In the face of scarce resources, technologies that produce relatively large benefits at a low cost have greater worth than technologies that offer few benefits and high costs. Spurred by the trends toward cost containment and evidence-based medicine, the number of cost-effectiveness evaluations of medical technologies—preventive, behavioral, diagnostic, reparative, or pharmaceutical—in the published literature has skyrocketed over the past two decades (Gold et al. 1996). Specific standards for conducting cost-effectiveness studies of medical technologies have emerged to ensure quality and adherence to fundamental elements of the methodology (Gold et al. 1996). Because new technologies are always being created, cost-effectiveness studies will likely be a major area of evaluation for many years to come.

This textbook is designed to provide a practical foundation for conducting evaluations in these arenas. The concepts and methods are similar to those found in the evaluation of social programs but have been customized for public health and medical care. Evaluation itself is a process conducted in a political context and composed of interconnected steps; another goal of this book is to help evaluators navigate them in health settings. A customized, reality-based treatment of health program evaluation should improve learning and ultimately may produce evaluations that are both practical and useful.

SUMMARY

At its core, evaluation entails making informed judgments about a program's worth, ultimately to promote social change for the betterment of society. Unprecedented growth in health programs and the health care system over the past three decades is largely responsible for the development of health program evaluation. Other forces contributing to the growth of the field include the increasing importance of accountability, escalating health care costs and the growth of managed care, scarce resources, greater emphasis on prevention and evidence-based medicine, reliance on demonstration projects, and a large increase in health care administrators, who are major consumers of evaluation information. Because many of these trends will continue in the 21st century, so will interest in the evaluation of health programs, health services, and the performance of the health care system. To perform any one of these three types of program evaluations, an evaluator completes a process composed of well-defined steps. In the next chapter, the elements of the evaluation process are described.

LIST OF TERMS

Evaluation

Health care system

Health program

Health services

Program

STUDY QUESTIONS

1. What is the purpose of health program evaluation?

2. What are the two fundamental questions of program evaluation?

3. How is the worth of a health program determined?

4. What are three factors that contributed to the growth of health program evaluation over the past three decades? Why are they important?

5. What are the major types of health program evaluation, and what are their relationships (if any) to each other?

CHAPTER 2

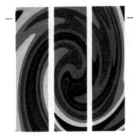

The Evaluation Process as a Three-Act Play

Performing a health program evaluation involves more than just the application of research methods. Evaluation is a *process* composed of specific steps designed to produce information about a program that is relevant and useful for decision makers, managers, program advocates, health professionals, and other groups. Understanding the steps and their interconnections is just as fundamental to evaluation as knowledge of the quantitative and qualitative research methods for assessing program performance.

There are two basic perspectives on the evaluation process. Based on the rational model of decision making, evaluation is a technical activity, where research methods from the social sciences are applied in an objective manner to produce information about program performance for use by decision makers (Faludi 1973; Veney and Kaluzny 1998). In practice, however, the evaluation of health programs rarely conforms to the rational model. Because politics is how we attach values to facts in our society, politics and values are inseparable from the evaluation of health programs (Palumbo 1987; Weiss 1972). Consequently, evaluations are conducted in a political context where a variety of interest groups compete for decisions in their favor. Completing an evaluation successfully depends greatly on the evaluator's ability to navigate this political terrain. In this chapter, the political nature of the evaluation process is depicted as a "three-act play." The remaining chapters of the book are organized around each act of the play.

EVALUATION AS A THREE-ACT PLAY

Drawing from Chelimsky's earlier work (1987), I use the metaphor of a "three-act play" to describe the political nature of the evaluation process. The play has a variety of actors and interest groups, each having a role, and each entering and exiting the political "stage" at different points in the evaluation process. Evaluators are one of several actors in the play, and it is critical for them to understand their role if they are to be successful. The evaluation process itself generates the plot of the play, which varies from program to program and often has moments of conflict, tension, suspense, quiet reflection, and even laughter as the evaluation unfolds.

Table 2.1 presents the three acts of the play, which correspond to the basic steps of the evaluation process (Andersen 1988). The play begins in the political realm with "Act I: Asking the Question," where evaluators work with decision makers to define the questions that the evaluation will answer about a program. This is the most important act of the play, for if the questions do not address what decision makers truly want to know about the program, the evaluation and its findings are more likely to have little value and use in decision making. In Act II, the political realm is left behind, to some degree, and research methods are applied to answer the questions raised in Act I. Finally, in Act III, the process re-enters the political realm, and the answers to the evaluation and policy questions provide insights that influence decision making and policy about the program.

Act I has two parts, or "scenes." In Scene 1, the evaluation process begins when decision makers authorize the evaluation of a program. In general, decision makers, program managers, and other groups may want to evaluate a program for *overt* and *covert* reasons (Weiss 1972, 1998a). Overt reasons are explanations that conform with the rational model of decision making and are generally accepted by the public (Weiss 1972, 1998a). In this context, evaluations are conducted to make decisions about whether to

▸ Continue or discontinue a program

▸ Improve program implementation

▸ Test the merits of a new program idea

▸ Compare the performance of different versions of a program

▸ Add or drop specific program strategies or procedures

TABLE 2.1   Evaluation as a Three-Act Play

ACT I: Asking the Question

Scene I:	Development of a policy question
Scene II:	Translation of the policy question into an evaluation question

ACT II: Answering the Question

Scene I:	Development of an evaluation design to answer the question
Scene II:	Development of the methods to carry out the design
Scene III:	Conducting the evaluation

ACT III: Using the Answers in Decision Making

Scene I:	Translation of evaluation answers back into policy language
Scene II:	Development of a dissemination plan for evaluation answers
Scene III:	Use of the answers in decision making and the policy cycle

▶ Implement similar programs elsewhere

▶ Allocate resources among competing programs

Because Act I occurs in the political arena, covert reasons for conducting evaluations also exist (Weiss 1972, 1998a). Decision makers may launch an evaluation to

▶ Delay a decision about the program

▶ Escape the political pressures from opposing interest groups, each wanting a decision about the program favoring its own position

▶ Provide legitimacy to a decision that already has been made

▶ Promote political support for a program by evaluating only the good parts of the program and avoiding or covering up evidence of program failure

Whether a program is evaluated for overt or covert reasons may depend on the viewpoint of the different actors and groups in the play (Shortell and Richardson 1978). The *funding agency* may want to evaluate a program to determine its cost-effectiveness and discover whether the program has any unintended, harmful effects. The *organization* that runs the program may be interested in an evaluation to demonstrate to interest groups that the program works, justify past or future expenditures, gain support for expanding the program, or simply satisfy reporting requirements imposed by the funding agency.

Program administrators may support an evaluation because it can bring favorable attention to a program that they believe is successful, which may help them earn a promotion later on. Administrators also may use an evaluation as a mechanism for increasing their control over the program, or to gather evidence to justify expanding the program, or to defend the program against attacks from interest groups that want to reduce or abolish it. *Program evaluators* may want to conduct an evaluation for personal reasons, such as to earn an income or to advance their careers. Alternatively, the evaluator may sympathize with a program's objectives and see the evaluation as a means toward promoting them. Other evaluators are motivated to evaluate because they want to contribute to the discipline's knowledge by publishing their findings or presenting them at conferences.

Finally, the *public* and its various interest groups may endorse evaluations for accountability, or to ensure that tax dollars are being spent on programs that work. Alternatively, interest groups that either support or oppose the program may advocate for an evaluation, with the hope of using "favorable" results to promote their point of view in Act III of the evaluation process. The public also may support evaluations because they are the source of information—in the mass media, on the Internet, in medical journals, and elsewhere—about the advantages and disadvantages of preventive and therapeutic technologies in medicine and dentistry. Given public concerns about the performance of managed care organizations, the public also is interested in evaluations that help them choose their sources of health care and health insurance.

In Scene 1 of Act I, decision makers and other groups develop one or more policy questions about the program (see Chapter 3). A policy question is a general statement indicating what "decision makers" want to know about the program. Decision makers can include the funding agency, the director of the organization that runs the program, the program's manager and staff, outside interest groups, and the program's clients. Together, they constitute the "audience" of the play, and the objective of the evaluation is to produce results that will be used by at least some members of a program's audience.

Although decision makers may authorize an evaluation of a health program for a variety of reasons, many evaluations are performed to answer two fundamental questions: Did the program succeed in achieving its objectives? and Why is this the case? For some programs, however, decision makers may want to know more about the program's implementation than its success in achieving its objectives. For example, questions about achieving objectives may be premature for new programs that are just finding their legs, or when decision makers want to avoid information about the program's successes and failures, which may generate controversy downstream in Act III of the evaluation process. In these and other cases, the basic policy question becomes "Was the program implemented as intended?" As the number of decision makers from different interest groups increases, so can the number of policy questions about the program. When a program addresses a controversial, political issue, heated debates may arise among decision makers and interest groups about what questions should and should not be asked about the program. Evaluators can play an important role when they facilitate communication among the decision makers and interest groups to help them form a consensus about what policy questions to ask about the program. In addition to moderating the discussions, evaluators also can be active participants and pose their own policy questions for decision makers to consider. If the program is already up and running, evaluators can support the discussions by providing descriptive information about program activities that may help decision makers formulate questions or choose among alternative questions.

If the play is to continue, Scene 1 ends with one or more well-defined policy questions endorsed by decision makers and, in some contexts, by at least some interest groups. The play may end in Scene 1, however, if no questions about the program are proposed, or if decision makers cannot agree on a policy question or what the program is trying to accomplish (Weiss 1998a). For covert reasons, decision makers may place stringent limits on what questions can and cannot be asked when they want to avoid important issues, or possibly to cover up suspected areas of program failure. Under these conditions, evaluation findings may have little influence on people's views of the program, and consequently, there is little value in conducting the evaluation (Weiss 1998a).

Once one or more policy questions are developed, Scene 2 begins and the policy questions are translated into feasible evaluation questions. In Scene 2, the evaluator is responsible for translating a general policy question, such as "Does the program work?", into a more specific evaluation question, such as "Did the smoking prevention program reduce cigarette smoking behavior among adolescents between the ages of 13 and 15?" To ensure that the evaluation will produce information that decision makers want in Act III of the play, decision makers should review the evaluation questions and formally approve them before advancing to the next act of the play.

In Scene 2, the evaluator also is responsible for assessing the feasibility of designing an evaluation and collecting the data to answer the question. Before going ahead with the evaluation, the evaluator should confirm that adequate resources, including time and qualified staff (or consultants), exist to conduct the evaluation (Weiss 1998a). The evaluator should verify that data required for answering the questions are available or can be collected, and that a sufficient number of observations will exist for subsequent data analyses (see Chapter 7). The feasibility assessment also should confirm whether the program has matured and has established stable routines (Weiss 1998a). Stable programs are preferred because the reasons for program success or failure can be identified more readily than in unstable programs. With stable programs, evaluation findings based on data collected a year ago have a better chance of still being relevant today. In contrast, when a program is changing continually, the findings obtained at the end of the evaluation process may apply to a program that no longer exists. If no insurmountable obstacles are encountered and the evaluation appears to be feasible, the evaluator and the other actors in the play have a "green light" to proceed to the next act of the evaluation process.

In "Act II: Answering the Question," the evaluation is actually conducted. Evaluators apply research methods to produce information that answers the evaluation questions raised in the previous act. As the evaluation itself becomes the focus and dominates the play, the political issues in Act I assume minor roles as decision makers and interest groups await the findings of the evaluation.

Evaluations may be *prospective* or *retrospective*. In a prospective evaluation, the evaluation is designed *before* the program is implemented, as shown in Table 2.2. Prospective evaluations are ideal because a greater number of approaches can be considered for evaluating a program. With greater choice, evaluators have more flexibility to choose an approach with the most advantages and least disadvantages. In addition, evaluators have more freedom to specify the information they want to collect about the program and, once the program is implemented, to ensure that the information is actually gathered.

In contrast, retrospective evaluations are designed and conducted *after* a program has ended, and a smaller number of alternative approaches usually exist for evaluating such programs. Historical information about the program may exist in records and computer files, but the information may not be useful for answering key questions about the program. In retrospective evaluations, choice of design and availability of information are almost always compromised, which may limit what can be learned about the program.

TABLE 2.2   The Prospective Evaluation Process

1. Define the problem
   ▷ What is the problem?
   ▷ Why is it a problem?
   ▷ What are its attributes?
      ▷ Target population
      ▷ Needs assessments
2. Design a program and specify objectives to address the problem
3. Develop the program's intervention(s)
4. Design the evaluation
5. Implement the program
6. Conduct the evaluation
7. Disseminate findings to decision makers

In Scene 2, evaluators develop one or more *evaluation designs* to answer each evaluation question raised in Act I. There are two basic types of evaluation designs. *Impact evaluations* (also known as "outcome" or "summative" evaluations) address the first policy question and use experimental or quasi-experimental designs to estimate program effects (see Chapters 4 and 5). Experimental designs use randomization to determine whether observed outcomes are due to the program. In many programs, however, randomization is not possible because laws prohibit excluding groups from the program, logistics prevent random assignment to program and control groups, the evaluation is performed after the program ends, or for other reasons. In these cases, quasi-experimental designs (such as interrupted time series, regression discontinuity analysis, and nonequivalent control group designs) are often used to estimate program effects. In general, the greater the political controversy in Act I, the greater the importance of having a rigorous impact design that can withstand public scrutiny when the results of the evaluation are released to the public.

Evaluation of *program implementation*, which is also known as *process evaluation*, addresses the second basic policy question and attempts to explain why programs do or do not achieve their objectives by examining how they were implemented (see Chapter 6). Implementation evaluations typically are designed to answer the following questions:

▶ Was the program implemented as intended?

▶ Did the program reach its intended target group?

▶ What services did people in the program receive?

▶ Were people satisfied with the program's services?

▶ What is the average cost for each person who received the program?

To answer these and other kinds of questions, implementation evaluations use both quantitative methods (such as surveys and the abstraction of insurance claims) and qualitative methods (such as focus groups, personal observation, and interviews) to gather information about a program. When an impact evaluation is based on a quasi-experimental design, evidence from an implementation evaluation is useful for interpreting the impact results and deciphering whether the program or other forces accounted for program outcomes. Scene I culminates in an evaluation plan, which serves as a "blueprint" for organizing and performing the impact and implementation evaluations within a given budget and period of time.

In Scene 2, detailed methods are developed to carry out the design (see Chapters 7, 8, and 9). For example, if the evaluation plan requires a telephone survey of sampled program participants, in Scene 2 the sampling protocols would be developed and the telephone instrument would be constructed, pretested, revised, and readied for implementation in the field. Then, in Scene 3, the evaluation is actually conducted according to the plan. The evaluator collects and analyzes data in ways that produce specific answers to each evaluation question raised in Act I. On the basis of the evidence, the evaluator may formulate one or more recommendations for decision makers and other members of the play's audience to consider in the final act of the play.

In "Act III: Use of the Answers in Decision Making," the evaluation returns to the political realm, where findings are disseminated to the evaluation's audience (see Chapter 10). A central assumption is that evaluations have worth only when their results are actually used by decision makers to improve program performance, to formulate new policy, or for other purposes (Patton 1997; Rossi and Freeman 1993). Historically, however, the evidence indicates that this is often not the case (Rossi and Freeman 1993; Weiss 1972, 1998a). To encourage the use of evaluation findings, evaluators must translate the answers to the evaluation questions back into policy language for each policy question raised by decision makers and interest groups in Act I. Then, evaluators can develop formal dissemination plans to ensure that each interest group receives the information it wants about the program in a timely manner.

In the end, decision makers and other groups in the audience are more likely to use the answers if they played an active role in creating the policy and evaluation questions in Act I, reinforcing the circular nature of the play and the notion that upstream events can have downstream consequences for decision making (Shortell and Richardson 1978). As the play comes to a close, the results of an evaluation are not the final determination of a program's worth, which is ultimately a political decision based on the combination of facts and values. Findings can, however, provide public evidence about a program to reduce uncertainties and clarify the gains and losses that decisions might cause (Weiss 1972).

There are three important features of the play in health program evaluations. First, although the evaluation process is portrayed as a linear flow from Act I to Act III, the process is often circular between the acts. For example, the feasibility of an evaluation question in Act I may not be known fully until Act II, when the evaluation is designed in detail, and the evaluator discovers that the question cannot be answered because of incomplete data or for other reasons. In this case, the evaluator must return to Act I and reformulate the question or replace it with a new question. Similarly, reactions from the audience in Act III may indicate that data analyses in Act II missed important aspects of the program, and the evaluator must circle back to Act II to remedy the omission.

Second, evaluation is a "practice" and not a "cookbook." Just as physicians practice medicine in different ways, so do evaluators apply research methods in different ways to assess program performance. For any given program, many good designs may exist, but no perfect ones (Cronbach 1982; Rossi and Freeman 1993). Through daily practice, each evaluator develops his or her own "evaluation style" for working with other actors in the play, choosing among alternative designs, and traversing the three acts of the play.

Third, the three-act play is a general framework of the evaluation process, and different, customized versions of it can be found in public health. For example, public health practice consists of three core functions: assessment, policy development, and assurance, where evaluation is a component of the assurance function (see Table 2.3). The Centers for Disease Control and Prevention have developed a six-step framework for evaluating public health programs that contains the elements of the three-act play (Centers for Disease Control and Prevention [CDC] 1999). Similarly, Green and colleagues (Green and Kreuter 1999; Green and Lewis 1986) have developed a customized framework for evaluating health education and promotion programs that is based on the "precede-proceed" model, which contains the elements of the three-act play. Finally, Glasgow and associates (1999) propose their own RE-AIM framework for evaluating the public health impact of health promotion interventions in a popula-

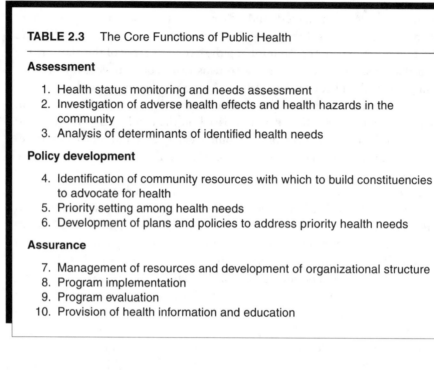

TABLE 2.3   The Core Functions of Public Health

Assessment

1. Health status monitoring and needs assessment
2. Investigation of adverse health effects and health hazards in the community
3. Analysis of determinants of identified health needs

Policy development

4. Identification of community resources with which to build constituencies to advocate for health
5. Priority setting among health needs
6. Development of plans and policies to address priority health needs

Assurance

7. Management of resources and development of organizational structure
8. Program implementation
9. Program evaluation
10. Provision of health information and education

tion of individuals. The framework contains both impact and implementation components of the three-act play, as well as an assessment of impacts on all members of the program's target population.

ROLE OF THE EVALUATOR

Just like all the other actors, the evaluator has a role to play that can greatly influence both the process and the outcomes of the evaluation. The role of the evaluator is not fixed and can vary from one health program to another. Although a variety of roles may exist in practice, four basic types can be defined.

In the three-act play described in the previous section, the evaluator has a *participatory role*, working closely with decision makers and other groups throughout the evaluation process (Cousins and Whitmore 1998). When the evaluator chooses to be an active participant, he or she also assumes responsibility for guiding decision makers and other groups through the evaluation process. The key advantage of the participatory role is that engaging decision makers in Acts I and II increases the likelihood that the evaluation will produce answers that decision makers want downstream in Act III.

The participatory role also has its disadvantages. The key danger is that evaluators may be co-opted by management and conduct studies that are too narrow and avoid important issues (O'Sullivan et al. 1985). Management co-optation may not be intentional; it may arise when administrators fear what may be found from the evaluation. As a consequence, the problem itself may be poorly defined, or the questions narrowly cast in Act I, to avoid exposing management's own poor performance in Act III.

O'Sullivan and colleagues (1985) illustrate this point using a case in which a North Carolina state agency ended its contracts to transport patients for renal dialysis. In response to the outcry from patient advocates, an evaluation was conducted to determine whether the cutback in transportation services had harmful consequences. The findings showed that patients continued to receive treatment and that death rates did not increase. The evaluators concluded that patients were not harmed seriously, and the agency's interest in the issue disappeared.

The evaluation, however, failed to examine the indirect impacts of the cutback (O'Sullivan et al. 1985). Because many patients had low incomes, they paid for transportation by cutting back on their food budgets and not buying needed medications. Because few patients drove themselves, family members had to take time off from work, reducing family earnings and increasing the emotional costs of being dependent on others. In short, the evaluation would have reached different conclusions if questions about changes in economic and emotional status also had been asked in Act I.

In contrast to the participatory role, evaluators also may play the role of the *objective researcher* (Weiss 1998a). The traditional role of the evaluator is to be an outside researcher who applies scientific research methods to produce an objective evaluation of the program. The evaluator values neutrality and consciously avoids becoming biased by the views of decision makers and other interest groups in the play. Some evaluators enjoy this role because of the autonomy, power, and authority that it gives them in the play. The chief advantage of the role is most visible when decision makers seek objective, unbiased information about a program, which they can use to address the competing demands from interest groups for decisions in their favor.

The detached role of the evaluator, however, also has its disadvantages. There is no consensus among evaluators and scientists about whether the application of research methods can ever be truly objective (Boudon and Bourricaud 1986). Evaluators are subject to the influence of their own beliefs and values as well as the social context of programs, which may influence what is and what is not observed about a program. Even though perfect objectivity is always an elusive goal, the objective evaluator can still strive for neutrality—that is, making unbiased observations about program performance that favor no individual or group.

By playing the role of outside researcher, the evaluator may become too "distant" from the program and fail to learn about what truly goes on in the program on a day-to-day basis. By emphasizing objectivity, the evaluator may rely too heavily on quantitative measures of program performance and miss qualitative information yielding different and valuable insights about the program. The role itself may create adversarial relationships with program staff, who may prefer working with evaluators who share their commitment to improving the program. Just as in the participatory role, if the objective researcher is responsive solely to questions raised by decision makers, he or she may be co-opted and miss important aspects of program implementation and performance.

In stark contrast to the objective researcher, evaluators also can play an *advocacy role* (Greene 1997). A basic premise of the role is that evaluators cannot be value neutral; therefore, advocacy is an inevitable part of their role. For evaluators, the question is not whether to take sides but whose side to be on (Becker 1967:239). In the advocacy role, the evaluator explicitly identifies his or her commitment to a set of values in the evaluation. Thus, if evaluators conclude that a health program improves health outcomes, which is consistent with their values, they are free to take a stance and persuade others to adopt it, provided they do not suppress evidence inconsistent with their conclusion (Cronbach 1987). The advantage of the role is that it increases the likelihood that recommendations from an evaluation will in fact be implemented. The disadvantage of the role is the possibility that evaluators will no longer be impartial in framing questions, in collecting evidence, and in being fair judges of the worth of the program.

In health program evaluation, evaluators either implicitly or explicitly play an advocacy role, because most health professionals share a value commitment to protecting the health of the public, promoting access to health care, delivering cost-effective services, and so forth (Greene 1997). As a common practice, therefore, advocacy evaluators should declare their value commitments and evaluate programs from a stance that promotes those values. By doing so, the evaluator advocates for *value positions* and not for *specific programs*, which can avoid at least some of the disadvantages of advocacy evaluation.

A fourth role for evaluators to play is to be the *coach* for evaluations conducted by community members (Weiss 1998a). Often known as empowerment evaluation (Fetterman et al. 1996), community members assume lead roles in planning, implementing, and evaluating their own programs. As a coach, the evaluator takes the role of offering help, advice, and guidance, and of promoting community ownership of the evaluation. The advantages of the role are found mainly in community empowerment and self-determination. Its major disadvantage is that community members may lack the knowledge and experience to conduct the evaluation, even with help from the coach, which may lead to inaccurate or incomplete findings.

One example of empowerment evaluation in public health is a 5-year program funded by the Centers for Disease Control and Prevention (CDC) to establish Urban Research Centers in Detroit, Seattle, and New York City (personal communication from Anissa Ham, CDC). The overall aim of the project is to find out "what works" to improve the quality of life of inner-city, impoverished populations. At each site, partnerships were created between the community, public health agencies, health systems, and academe. A participatory research process was followed to identify problems affecting the health of inner-city communities and to design, implement, and evaluate solutions to them. Community members prioritized local health problems, worked with the partners to identify what can be done about them, and were engaged in all phases of the evaluation process. Since 1995, the sites have addressed such issues as asthma prevention, access and quality in managed health care, family violence, HIV prevention, and immunizations.

In summary, evaluators can choose different roles to play in the evaluation process. The roles are not mutually exclusive, and an evaluator can shift between roles across the three acts in Table 2.1. The evaluator's choice of role typically is influenced by the funding source of the evaluation. When decision makers hire an evaluator from an outside agency to examine a health program, the decision maker may want the evaluator to play the role of the objective researcher. Similarly, evaluators in academia doing large-scale evaluations of health programs funded by government or foundations also may want to play this role. In fact, the Robert Wood Johnson Foundation historically has mandated that evaluations of its demonstration projects be performed by objective professionals who are not responsible for project implementation. In contrast, large health agencies with sufficient resources may hire their own evaluators to assess their health programs, and the agency may shape the role of the evaluator and, therefore, her or his relationships with other actors in the play.

ETHICAL ISSUES

In conducting evaluations, ethical issues often arise. Consider the following scenarios:

▶ In a process evaluation, staff report they have little say in program decisions, and the evaluator concludes that the program is too centralized. The director of the program refuses to distribute the final report unless the conclusion is changed (Palumbo 1987:26).

▶ The evaluator proposes a randomized design to determine the impacts of the program, but the director asks her to choose a less rigorous, quasi-experimental design to satisfy the demands of interest groups who are worried that some needy people will be denied the program in the randomized design (Morris 1998).

▶ The evaluator reports that a health program has no impacts, and the director of the program wants to suppress the report because she believes it may damage the program's future funding.

To help evaluators address these important dilemmas in their work, the American Evaluation Association has developed guiding principles to promote the ethical conduct of evaluations by its members. Five key principles are advanced, as summarized below (detailed guidelines are presented in American Evaluation Association 1995):

▶ *Systematic inquiry:* Evaluators should conduct systematic, data-based inquiries about whatever is being evaluated.

▶ *Competence:* Evaluators should provide competent performance to stakeholders.

▶ *Integrity/honesty:* Evaluators should ensure the honesty and integrity of the entire evaluation process.

▶ *Respect for people:* Evaluators should respect the security, dignity, and self-worth of the respondents, program participants, clients, and other stakeholders with whom they interact.

▶ *Responsibilities for general and public welfare:* Evaluators should articulate and take into account the diversity of interests and values that may be related to the general and public welfare.

Conflicts between the evaluator and the other actors often emerge in all three acts and contribute to the tension and drama of the play. In these difficult times, courage and character are personal qualities that can help evaluators uphold the ideals and values of their profession, and the guiding principles provide them with an important resource for doing so.

EVALUATION IN A CULTURAL CONTEXT

Reducing health disparities among Americans is a major goal of national health policy (U.S. DHHS 1991). The evidence indicates that people from some racial and ethnic minority groups, older adults, and people with disabilities have a higher incidence of death and disease than other groups. In response, public and private organizations have launched a variety of programs to reduce health disparities across diverse cultural groups (Lee and Estes 1994), defined by race and ethnicity, country of origin, religion, disability, age, gender, or sexual orientation (Lima and Schust 1997). Just as health programs must be customized to health beliefs, values, and practices of each culture, so must evaluations also consider these factors in each act of the play.

The importance of culture is illustrated by attempts to reduce cigarette smoking among Native Americans. Although smoking has declined for most racial groups, cigarette use among Native Americans has increased more than 40% ("Curbing Native American smoking" 1998). Reducing cigarette smoking among Native Americans is difficult because of their historical regard of tobacco as a sacred gift and its central place in Indian culture. Programs to reduce smoking or achieve other health objectives in a cultural group demand evaluations that reflect and respect the group's culture. This appreciation of culture may be achieved by

- Including members of the cultural group as full participants in all acts of the play

- Ensuring that the values and traditions of the culture are taken into account in the design of the program as well as the evaluation

- Considering cultural factors in the choice of measures and data collection protocols

- Having members of the cultural group interpret the findings of the evaluation and develop recommendations for decision makers.

On the basis of the guiding principles of the American Evaluation Association, evaluators have a responsibility to understand the role of culture in evaluation if they are to practice in an ethical manner (McDowell 1992).

SUMMARY

The evaluation process consists of three basic steps. The first step occurs in the political realm, where evaluators work with decision makers and other groups to define the questions that the evaluation will answer about the program. In the second step, the evaluation is conducted to produce information that provides the answers to the questions. In the third step, the evaluation returns to the political realm, and findings are disseminated to decision makers, interest groups, and other constituents. The metaphor of a three-act play is used to illustrate how political forces shape the evaluation process and the role of the evaluator. Ethical issues can arise in all acts of the play, and to meet these challenges, the American Evaluation Association (AEA) has developed guiding principles to promote the ethical conduct of evaluations. Because health programs often are created to reduce health disparities across cultural groups, evaluations also must consider cultural factors in their design and conduct. Act I of the play begins in the next chapter, which describes how to develop evaluation questions.

LIST OF TERMS

Core functions of public health

Cultural context of evaluation

Ethics of evaluation

Evaluation process

Formative evaluation

Guiding principles of the AEA

Impact evaluation

Outcome evaluation

Process evaluation

Program implementation

Rational decision making

Roles of the evaluator

Summative evaluation

1. What are the three basic steps of the evaluation process, or the three-act play? How does politics influence the evaluation process? What are some of the overt and covert reasons for conducting evaluations? Which actors in the play may desire an evaluation, and for what reasons?

2. What are the two basic types of evaluation? How are they interrelated with each other?

3. An evaluator can adopt different roles in the play. What are these roles, and can an evaluator play more than one role at the same time?

4. What ethical dilemmas often confront evaluators? How can the guiding principles for evaluators help resolve these dilemmas in the field?

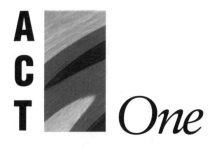

ACT One

ASKING
THE
QUESTION

CHAPTER 3

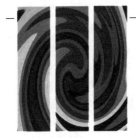

Developing Evaluation
Questions

The evaluation process begins in "Act I: Asking the Question," and the evaluator's goal is to develop one or more questions about the health program. Specifying clear, well-defined evaluation questions is the most important part of the play because the questions will direct the design and conduct of the evaluation in Act II and, hence, the answers obtained and disseminated in Act III.

Evaluators can identify questions by asking decision makers and interest groups what they want to know about the program, and then translating their responses into specific evaluation questions. In some cases, decision makers may not have a clear idea about what questions to ask, or they may simply delegate this task to the evaluator. In other cases, decision makers may ask only politically "safe" questions that, when answered and disseminated in Acts II and III, will not stir up controversy about the program. Regardless of the context, the evaluator's goal is to build in-depth knowledge about the health program and, based on this understanding and the application of evaluation principles, to pose questions that *should* be asked about the program.

This chapter describes how to develop evaluation questions through four basic steps: (a) specify program theory, (b) specify the program objectives, (c) translate program theory and objectives into evaluation questions, and (d) select key questions to answer in Act II of the evaluation process.

STEP 1: SPECIFY PROGRAM THEORY

In general, programs succeed or fail largely based on the accuracy of the underlying assumptions about how they are supposed to work. These assumptions may be divided into two groups: the program's *theory of cause and effect* and the program's *theory of implementation* (Chen 1990; Chen and Rossi 1983; Cole 1999; Lipsey 1993; Pressman and Wildavsky 1984; Reynolds 1998; Shortell 1984; Weiss 1995, 1997).

A program's theory of cause and effect is the underlying logic explaining why a program will cause specific outcomes. These causal connections often are captured by "if-then" statements about the program: "If I do X (the program), then Y (the desired outcome) will result," presented graphically, "$X \rightarrow Y$."

Programs also have a theory of implementation, which defines the strategy for implementing a program in the field (Shortell 1984). Most health programs can be implemented in different ways, or through different strategies. A program's performance is determined partly by the strategy for implementing the program in the field and partly by whether the strategy is actually implemented as intended.

Although somewhat oversimplified, the idea is that whether a program succeeds or fails depends on whether its theory of cause and effect and theory of implementation are sound, as shown in Table 3.1. Programs are successful only when a sound theory of cause and effect and theory of implementation combine to produce intended outcomes (cell 1). In contrast, programs may fail to achieve intended outcomes because of (a) faulty assumptions in the program's underlying theory of cause and effect (cell 2); (b) failure of the program to be implemented as intended, or if implemented as intended, choice of the wrong strategy of implementation (cell 3); or (d) both (cell 4).

To illustrate program theory, Figure 3.1 presents the theory of cause and effect for "A Healthy Future," a demonstration project for Medicare enrollees at Group Health Cooperative of Puget Sound (Patrick et al. 1999). Recognizing the potential benefits of prevention and Medicare's lack of coverage for preventive services, in 1987 Congress mandated demonstrations (known as the COBRA demonstrations) to assess the cost-effectiveness of delivering preventive services to Medicare enrollees in health maintenance organizations and fee-for-service settings (Grembowski et al. 1993). Group Health Cooperative of Puget Sound, a health maintenance organization (HMO), was one of six sites to conduct the demonstration.

In 1989, 5,012 Medicare beneficiaries in four medical centers at Group Health Cooperative were invited to participate in the demonstration, and 2,558

TABLE 3.1   Reasons for Program Success and Failure

		Theory of Program Cause and Effect	
		Sound	Faulty
Theory of Program Implementation	Sound	1. Program success	2. Causal logic problem
	Faulty	3. Implementation problem	4. Program failure

enrollees (51%) consented to do so. About half of the consenting adults ($N = 1,282$) were randomized to the intervention group that received an annual package of preventive services for 2 years, and the other half were randomized to the control group ($N = 1,276$) receiving usual care. The package of preventive services consisted of a health risk assessment, health promotion and disease prevention services from a nurse and the patient's physician, and health promotion classes. A computer program was developed to determine the health risks of enrollees from survey information collected at baseline. After the health risk assessment, intervention participants received a 90-minute health promotion visit from a trained nurse in the medical center where they usually received care (see Table 3.2). All participants received counseling to improve exercise behavior, to change diets to reduce fat and increase fiber, to complete advance directives and housing plans, and to consider insurance for long-term care. Following the visit, health promotion classes were offered in three areas. The disease prevention component consisted of a 60-minute visit with the enrollee's physician and nurse (see Table 3.2). Physical exams were conducted, health promotion plans were reviewed, and participants were encouraged to participate in classes. Medicare paid Group Health Cooperative $186.03 for each Medicare enrollee who received the full package of preventive services in each year of the 2-year demonstration, plus $20 for each baseline health risk assessment conducted for enrollees in the intervention group.

The demonstration's theory of cause and effect posits that compared to Medicare enrollees receiving usual care, the package of preventive services will increase self-efficacy and autonomy in decision making among those in the intervention group, which should lead to beneficial changes in health behavior that reduce health risks of older adults. These changes, in turn, would slow the natural decline in health and quality of life for older adults in the intervention

Figure 3.1. Theory of Cause and Effect for "A Healthy Future"

SOURCE: Reprinted from Patrick DL, et al. "Cost and Outcomes of Medicare Reimbursement for HMO Preventive Services." *Health Care Financing Review* 1999; 20(4):27.

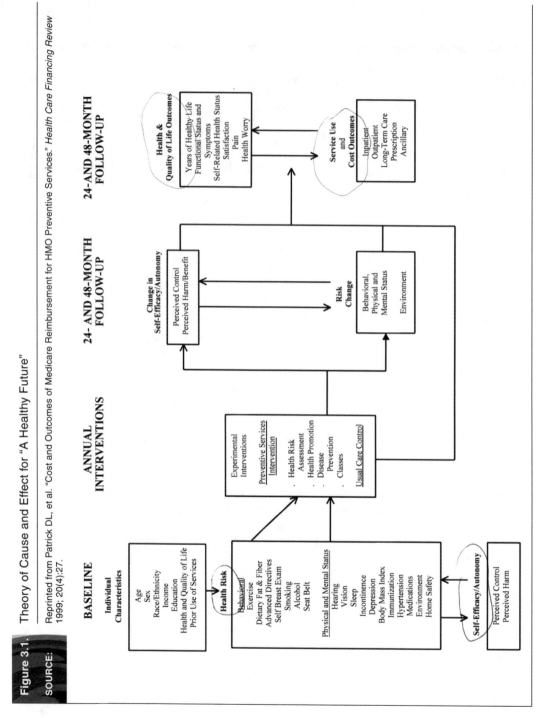

TABLE 3.2   "A Healthy Future" Demonstration's Health Promotion and Disease Prevention Services

Health Promotion Services (90-minute nurse visit)	Disease Prevention Services (35-minute physician visit and 25-minute nurse visit)	Health Promotion Classes
Exercise	Physical exam and laboratory	Exercise orientation
Nutrition (fat and fiber)	Height	Planning ahead
Planning ahead (living wills, power of attorney, housing plans)	Weight	Life satisfaction/ mental health
	Rectal Exam	
Mental health (depression, stress, sleep disturbance)	Stool hemoccult	
	Hematocrit	
Hearing impairment	Total cholesterol/HDL	
Review of medications	For women only	
Hypertension	Breast exam	
Alcohol use	Pelvic exam	
Smoking	Pap smear	
Breast cancer screening		
Home safety (falls)	Immunizations	
Vision	Influenza	
	Diptheria-tetanous	
	Pneumococcus	
	Counseling/Follow-up	
	Depression	
	Sleep/stress	
	Review of medications	
	Hypertension	
	Incontinence screening	
	Exercise	
	Planning ahead	
	Nutrition	
	Alcohol use	
	Smoking	
	Evidence of falls	
	Vision	
	Seat belt use	

group, resulting in lower utilization and costs of health services. In addition, the physical examination, laboratory, and immunization services in the disease prevention visit also would produce similar benefits.

A central concept of Bandura's social learning theory, self-efficacy refers to individuals' assessments of their effectiveness or competency to perform specific behaviors successfully (Bandura 1992; Grembowski et al. 1993). Several studies have shown that preventive self-efficacy, or an individual's perceptions of his or her ability to perform specific health behaviors, greatly influences actual health behavior and health status.

Autonomy is a global concept related to notions of control or sense of control over one's environment and life. A goal of the intervention was to promote autonomy in making health decisions, which should lead to greater participation in decisions concerning life-sustaining treatment and potentially lead to lower costs of care during the final months of life. In the program's theory of cause and effect, self-efficacy and autonomy are *mediating variables*; they are the mechanisms that explain why the package of preventive services will result in more healthy lifestyles, better health, and fewer doctor and hospital visits (Baron and Kenny 1986; Hallam and Petosa 1998; Weiss 1997).

The program's theory of implementation is to deliver a package of preventive services to Medicare enrollees in the intervention group, and the strategy for doing so was to provide the preventive services through individual appointments with nurses and physicians, as well as through health promotion classes. To carry out this strategy, five basic activities were performed, as shown in Figure 3.2. Providers were recruited in four medical centers at Group Health Cooperative. Health promotion materials and study protocols were developed for the intervention group, and providers attended orientation classes about the study and prevention for older adults. Next, Medicare enrollees in the four medical centers were recruited, and participants completed a baseline risk assessment. Third, the first round of preventive services was delivered through health promotion and disease prevention visits and classes. Fourth, as part of the health promotion visit, participants developed a formal plan to change one or more risky health behaviors. Last, in the second year of the demonstration, another round of preventive services was offered to participants, with additional work on continuing areas of health risk. The expected, immediate outcomes for the intervention group were improvements in self-efficacy and reductions in risky behaviors, as well as high satisfaction with the preventive service package.

Clearly, other implementation strategies are also possible. For example, at the demonstration site in Los Angeles, a different strategy was chosen. The package of preventive services was provided to older adults at a health fair held at a large conference center, which adults could attend on 1 of 3 days (Schweitzer et al. 1994). The strategy's key assumptions are that a health fair can bring a large number of people and health professionals together at one time, and that people can learn a lot about their health and enjoy themselves,

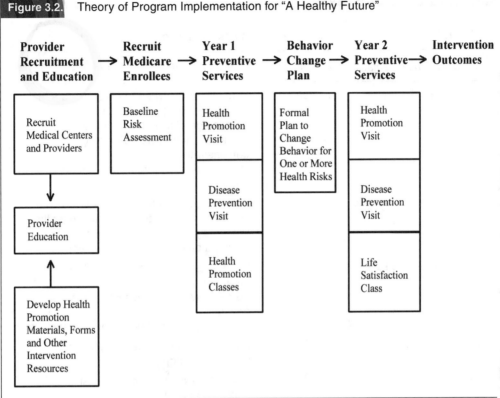

Figure 3.2.   Theory of Program Implementation for "A Healthy Future"

which may reinforce learning and encourage behavior change (Di Lima and Schust 1997). Even though the Seattle and Los Angeles sites had similar theories of cause and effect and similar preventive services, the different strategies for implementing the program could produce very different results.

The second part of the theory of implementation is whether the program was actually implemented as intended. To assess whether the demonstration project was implemented as intended, performance measures must be developed for each component of the program's theory of implementation, and the evaluation must collect data to track performance in each component. Table 3.3 presents examples of performance measures for each component of the demonstrations's theory of program implementation in Figure 3.2. For example, about 90% of adults in the intervention group received the intervention in the first year, and about 83% received the intervention in the second year, indicating that the group's exposure to the intervention was high.

TABLE 3.3   Examples of Performance Measures for Implementing "A Healthy Future"

Theory of Implementation Component	Examples of Performance Measures
Provider recruitment and education	▷ Percentage of invited medical centers that participated in the demonstration ▷ Percentage of invited physicians in the medical centers who participated in the demonstration ▷ Percentage of providers who attended orientation classes
Recruitment of Medicare enrollees	▷ Percentage of invited enrollees who consented to participate in the demonstration ▷ Percentage of participating enrollees completing a baseline risk assessment
Year 1 preventive services	▷ Percentage of enrollees with a health promotion visit ▷ Percentage of enrollees with a disease prevention visit ▷ Percentage of enrollees attending each class
Behavior change plan	▷ Percentage of enrollees with a formal behavior change plan
Year 2 preventive services	▷ Percentage of enrollees with visits (as indicated above) ▷ Percentage of enrollees with visits in both years 1 and 2

Both parts of a program's theory of implementation can affect the program's outcomes. The characteristics of persons and the features of program implementation that are thought or known to be associated with outcomes are called *moderating variables* (Weiss 1997). For example, gender and exposure to the program are moderating variables. A program may find that females do better than males, or adults who attend health promotion classes have a greater reduction in health risks than adults who do not attend classes.

Other examples of program theory exist in the literature. The Child and Adolescent Trial for Cardiovascular Health (CATCH) is a multisite, school-based intervention to reduce children's risk for heart disease by changing dietary patterns and physical activity (Luepker et al. 1996; McGraw et al. 1996). Similar to the Medicare study, the program's theory of cause and effect is based on social cognition theory: If the program causes changes in psychosocial factors (a mediating variable), such as self-efficacy in performing in healthy behaviors, they would lead to changes in risk behavior, which, in turn, would reduce serum cholesterol and, therefore, the threat of heart disease. The program's theory of implementation for its classroom component is shown in Figure 3.3. The model posits that teacher characteristics and training/support have direct effects on implementation—all moderating variables, which, in turn, influence both student participation and student outcomes, along with other factors. The implementation evaluation conducted by McGraw and her colleagues did not support the model as drawn in Figure 3.3. They found that *both* teacher and implementation characteristics had direct effects on student outcomes, and teacher characteristics did not affect implementation.

Another example is the large, community-based program to reduce lead poisoning in children living in low-income, dilapidated housing in New York City in 1970 (President and Fellows of Harvard College 1975). The problem affected primarily young children who ate chips of lead-based paint that peeled from tenement walls. To reduce children's exposure to paint chips, the city launched an ambitious program to screen 120,000 children for lead poisoning. If a child's blood lead level was high, the child's apartment was inspected, and if evidence of lead exposure was detected, wallboard was erected to prevent further exposure. The program's theory of implementation is illustrated in Figure 3.4. Although the incidence of lead poisoning decreased 80% in 3 years, the installation of wallboard did *not* cause the reduction. Instead, as a result of the wide-scale screening and publicity about the program, parents monitored their children's behavior more diligently, taking paint chips away when their children picked them up. In short, the program's theory of cause and effect, which assumed that children's exposure to lead paint would be reduced by house repairs, had an important omission. The program worked as intended but not for the reasons defined in its underlying theory of cause and effect.

In summary, mediating and moderating variables help explain the relationship between the program and its outcomes. Mediating variables relate to the program's theory of cause and effect and define the mechanisms explaining how the program causes observed outcomes. Moderating variables relate to the program's theory of implementation and define how the characteristics of people or the program's implementation are associated with outcomes.

Program theory has a number of important uses in the evaluation process. In Act I, program theory can help evaluators formulate questions about the program by increasing their understanding of how the program is supposed to achieve its objectives (Grembowski 1984). For example, a local health depart-

Figure 3.3. Conceptual Model for Process Evaluation of the Child and Adolescent Trial for Cardiovascular Health (CATCH)

SOURCE: McGraw SA, et al. "Using Process Data to Explain Outcomes: An Illustration from the Child and Adolescent Trial for Cardiovascular Health." *Evaluation Review*, 1996; 20(3):294. © Copyright 1996 by Sage Publications, Inc. Reprinted by permission of Sage Publications, Inc.

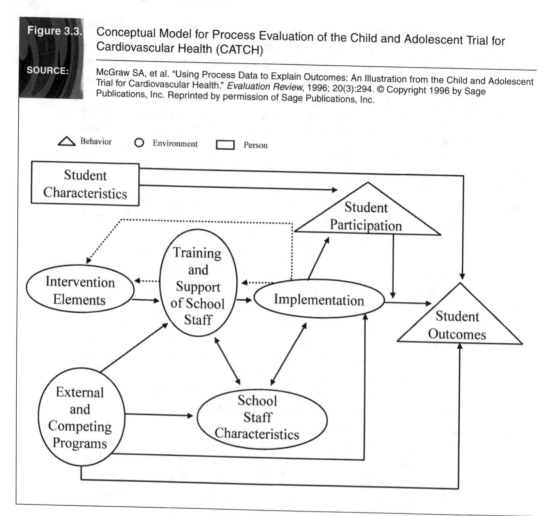

ment may decide to develop a smoking cessation program to reduce low birth weight among low-income, pregnant women (Windsor et al. 1988). Sheehan (1998) has examined the associations between stress, addictive behaviors (smoking and alcohol consumption), and low birth weight among 5,295 low-income, inner-city women in Hartford, Connecticut. Figure 3.5 presents his causal model, where the arrows indicate direct and indirect relationships between stress, addictive behavior, and low birth weight. Addictive behavior has a *direct effect* on low birth weight: The more a pregnant woman smokes or

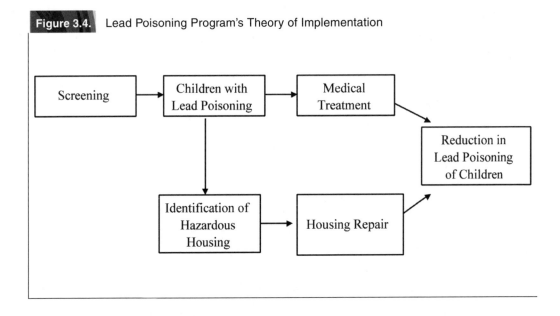

Figure 3.4. Lead Poisoning Program's Theory of Implementation

drinks alcohol, the lower the birth weight of her child. The standardized regression coefficient (.28) indicates how much change in low birth weight is produced by a standardized change in addictive behavior, controlling for other factors in the model (Blalock 1972; Namboodiri et al. 1975). Family stress and social support, in turn, have direct effects on addictive behavior, while economic stress has direct effects on family stress and social support. Thus, the three stress variables have *indirect effects* on low birth weight through their direct effects on addictive behavior.

If the smoking cessation program targets women with similar characteristics, the model may offer several insights about the program's theory of cause and effect. First, the model suggests that the program alone will likely reduce but not eliminate the problem of low birth weight. The model indicates that 90% of the variation in low birth weight is not explained by the variables in the model. In addition, the model indicates that both medical risks and addictive behavior have direct effects on low birth weight. Because the unexplained variance is large, and because the program may not reduce other risk factors, the program, by itself, will at best reduce but not eliminate low birth weight.

How much will the reduction be? The model suggests that the program's indirect effect on low birth weight will likely be smaller than .28. To illustrate this

Figure 3.5.   Stress and Low Birth Weight

SOURCE: Reprinted from Sheehan TJ. "Stress and Low Birth Weight: A Structural Modeling Approach Using Real Life Stressors." *Social Science and Medicine*, 1998; 47(10):1503-12, Figure 4. © Copyright 1998 Elsevier Science. Reprinted with permission from Elsevier Science.

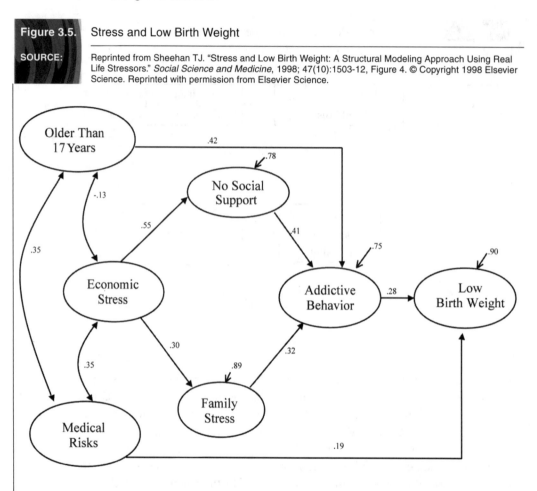

point, let's assume that the program reduces smoking by .25, and that the standardized regression coefficient measuring the program's effect on addictive behavior is .28. Then, the program's indirect effect on low birth weight is simply .25 × .28 = .07, assuming the program does not change the size of the association between addiction and low birth weight (Namboodiri et al. 1975).

Second, the model also may suggest how the program can be modified to increase its performance. For example, given that stress has a direct effect on addiction and indirect effects on low birth weight, the program may be more successful in reducing low birth weight if it also contains a stress reduction component targeted at one or more of the three sources of stress in the model.

Program theory also can help evaluators to identify important concepts of the program, which is important for deciding what should be measured about the program in the second act of the evaluation process. For example, if a health promotion program is designed to increase exercise by increasing participants' self-efficacy in the behavior, exercise self-efficacy is an important concept to measure in the evaluation (Hallam and Petosa 1998).

Program theory can help decision makers and interest groups develop policy and evaluation questions about the program. In the political process, decision makers and other interest groups often have different beliefs about how the program will produce expected benefits. Evaluators can discover these beliefs by asking them to sketch their own models of how the program works. By comparing their sketches, evaluators, decision makers, and interest groups can discover the differences and similarities in their underlying assumptions about how they expect the program to work. Through consensus meetings and workshops, evaluators can resolve differences that might exist to achieve a common view of a program's theory of cause and effect and theory of implementation. A common view of program theory is valuable because once everyone is working "from the same page," it is often easier to identify the key questions about the program in Act I and to develop evaluation designs for answering them in Act II.

STEP 2: SPECIFY PROGRAM OBJECTIVES

Once program theory is understood, the next step is to specify the program's objectives. Before an evaluation can be conducted, the evaluator must specify the criteria for judging whether the program is a success or failure. In most cases, the criteria are found in a program's objectives. The evaluator's goal is to define all of a program's objectives in ways that can be measured using clear, precise language that can be understood easily by all people in Act I of the evaluation process.

Most health programs have multiple objectives. For example, the ultimate objective of health education programs is to improve health status. To achieve this ultimate objective, however, several interrelated objectives must be achieved beforehand, as shown in Figure 3.6 (Mohr 1988; Suchman 1967). The material containing the health information must be printed and distributed to those who would benefit from it. Then, people who receive the material must actually read it and learn its salient messages, which, in turn, will lead to some type of change in behavior that ultimately improves or maintains health. This sequence of events is referred to as a *chain* or *hierarchy of objectives*, which may be divided into three levels: immediate, intermediate, and ultimate.

Table 3.4 presents immediate, intermediate, and ultimate objectives of the Medicare prevention program described earlier. At start-up, the focus was launching the program in the field, and the immediate objective was to recruit clinics, providers, and Medicare enrollees into the demonstration. Once those objectives were achieved, attention shifted to delivering the package of preventive services to the intervention group for 2 years and changing the self-efficacy and health behaviors of enrollees, which became the intermediate objectives of the program. After the 2-year intervention was completed, the end of hierarchy was reached: If the intermediate objectives were achieved and the intervention worked as intended, then the ultimate objectives of the program, slowing the decline in health and reducing the cost and utilization of health services, would be achieved.

Identifying a program's hierarchy of objectives is a valuable exercise because the hierarchy can help structure the evaluation of a program's implementation in Act II. In general, impact evaluations typically address whether a program has achieved its ultimate objectives. To find out whether a program was implemented as intended, implementation evaluations often examine whether the program's immediate and intermediate objectives were met, in essence verifying whether the means-ends relationship between each adjacent pair of objectives was satisfied (Suchman 1967). This approach to implementation evaluation will be described in more detail in Chapter 6.

The objectives of a program may be either clearly or poorly defined. In well-designed programs, objectives are clearly defined at all levels of the hierarchy. In other programs, only the ultimate objective of the program may be defined clearly, or program staff may have only a general notion of what the program is supposed to accomplish. In complex programs, it may be difficult to specify objectives in precise terms (Shortell and Richardson 1978). In other cases, objectives may not exist because program administrators worry they will set performance standards that the program cannot meet (Shortell and Richardson 1978). If clear program objectives do not exist, the evaluator must work with program staff and decision makers to define them. If program staff and decision makers cannot agree on what the program is supposed to accomplish, it will be virtually impossible to formulate evaluation questions about the program, and the best course may be to abandon the evaluation (Weiss 1972).

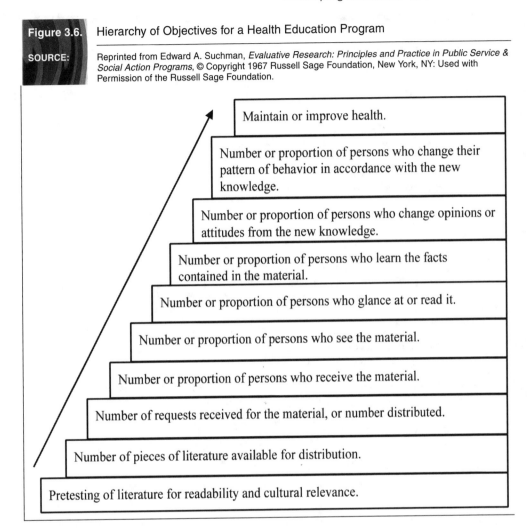

Figure 3.6.   Hierarchy of Objectives for a Health Education Program

SOURCE: Reprinted from Edward A. Suchman, *Evaluative Research: Principles and Practice in Public Service & Social Action Programs*, © Copyright 1967 Russell Sage Foundation, New York, NY: Used with Permission of the Russell Sage Foundation.

Maintain or improve health.

Number or proportion of persons who change their pattern of behavior in accordance with the new knowledge.

Number or proportion of persons who change opinions or attitudes from the new knowledge.

Number or proportion of persons who learn the facts contained in the material.

Number or proportion of persons who glance at or read it.

Number or proportion of persons who see the material.

Number or proportion of persons who receive the material.

Number of requests received for the material, or number distributed.

Number of pieces of literature available for distribution.

Pretesting of literature for readability and cultural relevance.

Specifying a program's objectives means writing a clear description of each one. This can be accomplished by identifying the parts of an objective, completing each part, and then arranging the parts to compose the objective. To illustrate this process, Table 3.5 presents an ultimate objective of the Medicare demonstration described earlier, and each part of the objective is broken down and described (Shortell and Richardson 1978).

In general, all programs are designed to *change* something—knowledge, beliefs, attitudes, or behaviors of individuals, organizations, communities, or

TABLE 3.4   Hierarchy of Objectives for "A Healthy Future," a Health Promotion and Disease Prevention Program for Medicare Enrollees[a]

I. Immediate objectives

   A. Clinic
      1. Recruit clinics and physicians
      2. Train providers and prepare for clinic implementation
   B. Subject
      3. Identify eligible Medicare enrollees
      4. Recruit and randomize enrollees

II. Intermediate objectives

      5. Identify participants' health risks in the intervention group
      6. Provide health promotion and disease prevention services and classes to participants in the intervention group in each year
      7. Increase behavior change plans among participants in the intervention group
      8. Increase health knowledge, self-efficacy, and healthy behaviors

III. Ultimate objectives

      9. Slow the decline in health
    10. Reduce utilization and costs

a. Different disciplines use different terms to describe program objectives. Some disciplines refer to the immediate objectives as "process" objectives and the intermediate objectives as "outputs." Other disciplines refer to ultimate objectives as impact objectives, while still others refer to them as outcome objectives. The three types of objectives in this table are intended to correspond to the terms used by other disciplines.

other social groups. An objective must contain the *source* of the change, which is usually the program itself, in this case the package of preventive services. An objective also must define *who* will change after receiving the program, *what* the program is going to change and by *how much*, and *when* the change is expected. For older adults, health status gradually declines after age 65 until death. The demonstration's package of preventive services was designed to slow this decline among Medicare participants in the intervention group by at least 50%. The objective does not specify explicitly how long the package of services will slow the decline in health, but when programs come to an end, their effects typically deteriorate over time.

Other guidelines are also helpful in writing clear objectives (Di Lima and Schust 1997; Shortell and Richardson 1978). First, an objective should contain a purpose *and* an end result. The purpose or aim of an objective defines what will be done; the end result describes what will be achieved. The statement "to

TABLE 3.5   Writing Program Objectives: An Example From the Medicare Demonstration

An ultimate objective of the Medicare demonstration	After 4 years, the preventive service package will reduce the decline of health status by 50% among Medicare enrollees in the intervention group
Source of change?	Preventive service package
Who will change?	Medicare enrollees who receive the preventive service package
What will change?	Health status of Medicare enrollees
When will it change?	After 4 years
How will it change?	Reduce the decline
How much will it change?	By 50%
How long will the change last?	Not specified

improve physicians' knowledge of the treatment of diabetes" is an example of an objective with an end result but no purpose or reference to the program. Adding text about the aim of the program resolves the problem: "to provide information about diabetes treatment to improve physicians' knowledge of diabetes treatment."

Second, an objective should contain only *one* purpose and *one* end result. If an objective contains two or more purposes or end results, it may be difficult to determine whether the objective was met later in the evaluation process. For example, the objective "to implement physical activity classes for older adults and provide transportation services for 10 adults per class" can create problems in the evaluation. The statement has two aims, implementing classes and providing transportation services. If one aim is met but the other is not, it will be difficult to conclude whether the objective is satisfied. A better strategy is to create two objectives, one for implementing classes and another for providing transportation.

Third, the end results of an objective should be observable and therefore measurable. Once an objective is specified in Act I of the evaluation process, evidence will be collected in Act II to determine whether the end result of the objective was achieved. An end result therefore must be a visible, tangible outcome that can be observed and measured in some way. For example, the objective "to provide free bicycle helmets to reduce head injuries among children in elementary schools" contains an observable end result, head injuries, that can be measured by reviewing the computer records of hospital emergency rooms in a community.

Fourth, objectives should contain "action-oriented" verbs that describe a behavior that can be observed. For example, "to *increase* immunizations" is an action-oriented statement of a behavior that can be observed. Other examples of action-oriented verbs include "to lower," "to improve," "to recruit," and "to implement." In contrast, "to *promote* immunizations" is a weaker and less specific statement. Other weaker, nonspecific verbs to avoid include "to understand," "to encourage," "to explore," and "to enhance."

Fifth, programs with multiple objectives should have a single statement for each objective. For example, the Medicare demonstration has two ultimate objectives, slowing the decline in health status and reducing the use and cost of health services, which require separate statements. In complex programs with multiple objectives, evaluators also should check whether one objective conflicts with another objective (Shortell and Richardson 1978). For example, a family medicine program in a medical school may have two clinical objectives: (a) to provide high-quality, continuous health care to the community; and (b) to refer patients to specialty departments to satisfy their teaching and research objectives. If the family medicine program aggressively refers patients to other departments, the program may not achieve its own goal of continuity in primary care. When conflicts between program objectives are detected in Act I, their impacts on program performance should be assessed later in Act II of the evaluation process.

STEP 3: TRANSLATE PROGRAM THEORY
AND OBJECTIVES INTO EVALUATION QUESTIONS

Once a program's theory and objectives are specified, the next step is to translate them into questions about the program to be answered in Act II of the evaluation process (Fink 1993). A central concern in most program evaluations is whether the program achieved its objectives. A program's hierarchy of objectives provides a structure for asking questions about a program's impacts and implementation.

Impact questions usually ask whether a program achieved its ultimate objectives. One approach to writing an impact question is simply to convert the ultimate objective into a question. For example, one of the ultimate objectives of the Medicare demonstration is presented below:

Ultimate Objective of Medicare Demonstration: After 4 years, the preventive service package will reduce the decline of health status by 50% among Medicare enrollees in the intervention group.

The ultimate objective can be converted directly into an impact question, as shown in Question A below. Question A, however, is quite specific. A "yes" answer is possible only if the program reduced the decline in health status *and* if the decline was 50% or more, relative to the control group. If the program reduced the decline in health status but by less than 50%, then the program did not achieve its ultimate objective, and the answer to Question A is "no." Impact questions therefore often omit specific performance standards and ask only if the program caused a change in the expected direction, as shown in Question B.

The Medicare demonstration also was expected to lower the utilization and cost of health services by the 4-year follow-up. Based on the demonstration's theory of cause and effect, if the preventive service package successfully reduced health risks and prevented illness, reductions in utilization and cost might follow. If the intervention was unsuccessful in reducing risky health behaviors or providing disease prevention services to older adults in the intervention group, the intervention would not have prevented illness in the intervention group, and therefore the intervention would not have reduced the utilization and costs of health care in the intervention group. In fact, the diagnostic tests given to the intervention group may have detected new medical problems, which could actually *increase* utilization and costs. Recognizing these interdependencies and contingencies among intermediate and ultimate objectives, Question C presents an impact question that does not specify the direction of change, if any, in utilization and costs.

Different Forms of Impact Evaluation
Questions for the Medicare Demonstration

A. Did the preventive service package reduce the decline in health status by 50% among Medicare enrollees after 4 years?

B. What is the effect of the preventive service package on the health status of Medicare enrollees at the 4-year follow-up?

C. What is the effect of the preventive service package on the utilization and cost of health services at each follow-up?

In a similar manner, questions about a program's implementation can be asked by converting a program's immediate and intermediate objectives into evaluation questions. Based on the Medicare demonstration's immediate and intermediate objectives in Table 3.4, examples of questions about the program's implementation are presented below.

Implementation Questions
About Immediate Objectives

D. What percentage of Medicare enrollees who were invited to participate in the demonstration consented to do so?

E. Were enrollees who participated different from those who did not enroll?

Implementation Questions
About Intermediate Objectives

F. What percentage of Medicare enrollees in the intervention group received the health promotion and disease prevention services from their providers or attended classes?

G. Of these enrollees, what percentage of adults received *each* health promotion and disease prevention service and attended each class? What percentage of enrollees developed a personal plan to change their health risks?

H. Did Medicare enrollees in the intervention group change their health behaviors at the 2-year follow-up? Did enrollees who developed a personal risk-reduction plan change their health behaviors more than enrollees who did not develop a plan?

I. What was the effect of the intervention on the health behaviors of Medicare enrollees at the 2-year follow-up?

Questions D through I address different groups of Medicare enrollees. Questions D and E address the entire sample of Medicare enrollees who were invited to participate in the demonstration. Questions F, G, and H, in contrast, address only Medicare enrollees in the intervention group; their aim is to find out whether the package of preventive services was actually delivered to enrollees in the intervention group. Question I, however, is an impact question; its aim is to determine whether the demonstration achieved its intermediate objective of changing the health behaviors of Medicare enrollees in the intervention group, relative to enrollees in the control group, as illustrated in the theory of cause and effect in Figure 3.1.

Program theory also may generate unique questions not connected to a program's hierarchy of objectives. Recall that a mediating variable of the Medicare demonstration is to increase the self-efficacy of intervention enrollees in performing specific health behaviors, and that none of the demonstration's objectives addresses this concept. In these cases, program theory is a source of evaluation questions. The impact question for the self-efficacy mediating variable may be written using the forms presented earlier, such as, Did the package of preventive services increase the self-efficacy of Medicare enrollees to perform specific health behaviors at each follow-up?

Finally, health programs may not work as expected, as explained in Table 3.1. A program may not affect outcomes, or it may actually have unintended, harmful consequences. If a health program is supposed to increase health status, then mortality is an unintended, negative outcome. Some health programs have unintended outcomes that are not anticipated at the start of implementation. For example, the national campaign to prevent domestic violence resulted in a variety of domestic-violence services, such as legal advocacy and hundreds of shelters for battered women, with the goal of reducing the number of women killed by their partners. Since 1976, the annual number of *women* killed by their partners has declined slightly; however, the number of *men* killed by their partners has dropped by more than two-thirds nationally. The disparity occurs because most domestic violence services aim to have women leave abusive relationships before violence escalates and women use deadly force to protect themselves, which also reduces the likelihood of male deaths (Masters 1999).

To identify unanticipated, unintended consequences, an evaluator should develop an in-depth understanding of the program by reviewing program records, talking with program managers and participants, talking with people who believe the program will fail, talking with people who are familiar with the program but are not responsible for achieving its objectives, brainstorming with other program evaluators, and examining the outcomes of similar programs implemented in other organizations (Shortell and Richardson 1978). As a "safety check," impact evaluations of health programs always should have one or more questions about whether the program had harmful consequences.

STEP 4: SELECT KEY QUESTIONS

If several questions are posed about a program, which ones should the evaluation address? For many programs, the basic options are to (a) focus on questions about the intermediate and ultimate objectives and conduct an impact evaluation, (b) focus on questions about the immediate and intermediate objectives and conduct an implementation evaluation, or (c) address both implementation and impact questions about the program. Unfortunately, there are no "gold standards" for choosing among these or other options; however, the factors described in the following paragraphs typically influence which questions to address or ignore (Shortell and Richardson 1978; Weiss 1998a).

Age of the Program

When a program is just starting, attention typically is concentrated on getting the program up and running in the field, establishing routines, and fixing problems as they arise. For new programs that have not achieved a steady state, an implementation evaluation with questions targeting the program's immediate and intermediate objectives can provide useful, timely information to improve the management of the program. Asking a question about the impacts of a new program is often premature because the program has not had sufficient time to achieve its ultimate objectives. If an impact evaluation is conducted of a new program and finds the program did not achieve its ultimate objectives, the results may be due simply to the timing of the evaluation rather than the performance of a mature program.

Budget

It may cost more to answer some questions than others. An evaluation may address only those questions that it can afford to answer.

TABLE 3.6   Guideline for Choosing the Type of Program Evaluation

Cause/effect relationship (does it work?)	Value/desirability of outcomes (is it worth it?)	
	Low	High
Unknown	1. Implementation evaluation	2. Impact evaluation
Known	3. Rigorous program evaluation	4. No formal evaluation (monitoring)

Logistics

In some programs, the data may not be available to answer a question, qualified personnel may not exist to conduct the evaluation, or there may not be enough time to answer a question and deliver the results to decision makers. In these contexts, it is often best to either abandon the question or modify it so that it can be answered with the available data and personnel by a given deadline.

Knowledge and Values

The choice of questions and, therefore, implementation or impact evaluation also may be influenced by what is known about the program's cause-and-effect relationships and the value or desirability of its outcomes, as shown in Table 3.6 (Shortell and Richardson 1978). As indicated in the rows of the table, little or extensive knowledge may exist about whether a program works and its theory of cause and effect. As the columns of the table show, preferences about the value or desirability of the program's outcomes may be classified as low or high. The cross-tabulation of the two dimensions creates four cells, each suggesting a different evaluation strategy.

In cell 1, little may be known about the program's cause-effect relationships, and little consensus may exist among individuals and groups about the value or desirability of the program's outcomes. For example, little agreement exists about whether "distant healing" (that is, an act of mentation performed to improve another person's health at a distance, such as prayer, mental healing, Therapeutic Touch, or spiritual healing) improves health, nor is there agreement that distant healing produces desirable outcomes (Astin et al. 2000). Reliance on prayer may have adverse outcomes for ill people, and anecdotal evidence suggests that Therapeutic Touch has negative side effects. In these cases, implementation evaluations may increase understanding of how the program works, which may help decision makers judge the desirability of the program and its outcomes. In Therapeutic Touch, for example, a useful approach is simply to document what the intervention consists of, who receives it and for what medical problems, whether formal protocols exist and are actually followed in practice, and whether patients are satisfied with the treatment. If this information indicates that implementation was satisfactory, and if outcomes are perceived as desirable, an impact evaluation targeted at the most common uses of the procedure might be warranted.

In cell 2, little is known about whether the program works, but most groups hope that it does. Impact evaluations addressing the program's intermediate and ultimate objectives are warranted. This is also a good place to examine whether the program's underlying theory of cause and effect and theory of implementation are working as intended. That is, do the mediating variables in a program's theory of cause and effect have important effects on program outcomes? Or do other factors have a greater influence on program outcomes? Similarly, do the linkages in a program's hierarchy of objectives work as expected? Do moderating variables influence whether the program's intermediate objectives are achieved? Clearly, a wide variety of questions can be explored, particularly when there are few budget and logistical barriers to doing so.

In cell 3, good evidence exists about a program's cause-effect relationships, but people are unsure about the program's worth. In this context, the program may be steeped in controversy, and rigorous evaluation of all objectives is warranted to help decision makers make judgments about whether the program should continue. In cell 4, much is already known about a highly desirable program, and only ongoing monitoring of program activities is warranted.

Consensus

Another option is to choose simply those questions that decision makers, program staff, and other groups all agree on. In participatory evaluations, each participant may want the evaluation to examine one or more questions. The evaluator can work with the participants through one-on-one or group meetings to achieve a consensus about what objectives to evaluate. Alternatively, the evaluator may give more weight to questions raised by groups most committed to using the findings of the evaluation to improve the program. The approach's advantages are that it promotes group participation in the evaluation process and that it establishes a common set of expectations about what kind of information will be disseminated about the program in Act III. Its disadvantage is that in some cases groups cannot agree on what questions to ask, and consequently all questions are chosen to satisfy all the groups, which may not be feasible when budget, personnel, or time constraints exist. Another disadvantage is that groups may purposively avoid questions that, when answered, may threaten the survival of the program.

Result Scenarios

Another strategy is to choose questions that, when answered, will likely change the beliefs, attitudes, and behavior of decision makers, program managers and staff, or other groups (Patton 1997). For example, if the evaluation results indicate that a program had no impacts, would these results change the funding, operations, or other features of the program? What if the program had a beneficial impact—would that result lead to program expansion or other changes? Questions may be worth asking if their answers will likely change people's beliefs, attitudes, or behavior about the program.

Funding

All evaluations require resources from a funding organization, or sponsor. Another strategy is to choose only those objectives that the evaluation's sponsor wants to pay for. The advantage of this approach is that priorities are established quickly, and evaluators can move directly into Act II and carry out the evaluation. Its primary disadvantage is that the sponsor may not be interested in answering key questions about the program, thereby co-opting the evaluator into addressing only the sponsor's interests. In such cases, the evaluator can increase the worth of the evaluation by convincing the sponsor to widen the scope by asking more questions about the program.

Evaluation Theory and Practice

Although evaluators should not dictate what questions to ask, they have a professional responsibility to identify "critical questions" about a program that may be overlooked by decision makers, program managers, or other groups. Critical questions can be identified in at least three ways. First, through their education and experience, evaluators possess knowledge about what standard questions to ask in most programs, such as

▶ Does it work?

▶ How does it work?

▶ Why does it work?

▶ When does it work?

▶ For what groups does it work?

▶ Under what conditions does it work?

▶ What attributes make it work?

▶ How do benefits compare with costs?

▶ Can it be replicated?

When program administrators and decision makers cannot articulate questions on their own, the evaluator can stimulate their thinking by raising common questions posed in most evaluations of health programs.

Second, questions can be raised about which groups do or do not benefit from the program. When a health program provides services to diverse social groups, outcomes may differ by race, age, gender, income, or disability for a variety of reasons. Asking questions about disparities in program performance is a good way to determine whether program implementation should be modified to reduce them.

In some cases, an evaluator may discover important questions to ask in early reviews of the program. In Act I of the evaluation process, the evaluator's goal is to learn as much as possible about "what goes on" within the program. In doing so, the evaluator may develop key insights about the program that suggest one or more critical objectives are not being met. For example, an evaluator may be asked to examine the health outcomes of patients undergoing cardiac catheterization. A preliminary review of the data suggests that black and white patients with similar coronary risk have different catheterization rates, with white patients having higher rates than black patients (Schulman et al. 1999). It is entirely appropriate for the evaluator to examine whether access to surgical procedures is equitable across racial groups, even though the sponsor and other groups may not have raised this question.

In summary, there may be more questions asked about a program than can be answered, given limits on available time, money, personnel, or other resources. A key role of the evaluator is to work with decision makers, program managers, and other groups to identify the critical questions that can be answered with the available resources by a given deadline. By their nature, implementation evaluations typically have more questions than impact evaluations. Because the number of questions is directly correlated with the time and costs required to complete an evaluation, a reasonable number of questions should be asked, typically fewer than 5 questions for impact evaluations and 5-10 questions for an implementation evaluation, with or without impact questions.

Assessment of Fit

Once the program's theory, objectives, and evaluation questions are defined, the three elements should be assessed for "goodness of fit," as shown in Figure 3.7. If you have followed the four steps described in this chapter, a close fit should exist among the program's theory, objectives, and evaluation questions. For example, if the goal of the Medicare demonstration is to slow the decline in health status of older adults by increasing their self-efficacy and healthy behaviors, the evaluation questions should address each of these three elements of the demonstration's theory and objectives. In contrast, a question about Medicare enrollees' emergency room visits would not reflect a good fit because neither the demonstration's theory nor its objectives target emergency services. If a good fit does not exist among a program's theory, objectives, and evaluation questions, each link among the three elements in Figure 3.7 should be inspected and revised, and this review should be repeated until all three elements are consistent with each other. The cross-check is important because it provides evidence that the evaluation's questions are, in fact, grounded on the program's theory and objectives, and therefore are relevant to assessing the program's worth. After the cross-check is completed and a proper fit is obtained, the evaluation process

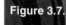 **Figure 3.7.** Assessment of Fit Among Program Objectives, Program Theory, Evaluation Questions, and Evaluation Methods

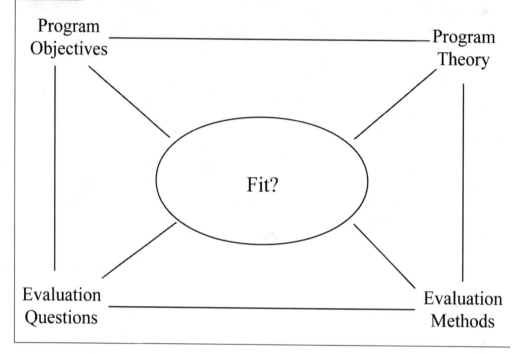

is ready to move forward into Act II, where evaluation methods are developed that also fit with the program's theory, objectives, and questions.

SUMMARY

The evaluation process is designed to answer questions that are raised about a program. In "Act I: Asking the Question," the evaluator's goal is to develop one or more questions by specifying program theory and objectives, translating both into evaluation questions, and, if too many questions exist, selecting questions that address key program issues. At the end of Act I, the evaluator should have a well-defined set of questions that most groups in the evaluation process can agree are worth asking. The evaluator's work now shifts from the political realm to the evaluation itself, where research methods are applied to collect information that answers each question raised in Act I. Act II opens in the next chapter with a discussion of how to design an evaluation to answer questions about a program's impacts.

_____LIST OF TERMS

Evaluation question   Moderating variables

Fit assessment   Program objectives

Hierarchy of objectives   Theory of cause and effect

Mediating variables   Theory of implementation

_____STUDY QUESTIONS

1. Programs typically have two underlying theories, a theory of cause and effect and a theory of implementation. Briefly describe each theory and how the two theories are related to each other.

2. Fleming and Andersen (1986) describe the Municipal Health Services program, which was designed to increase access to health care in low-income neighborhoods of selected U.S. cities. How would you diagram the program's theory of cause and effect? How would you diagram the program's theory of implementation?

3. What are three guidelines for writing evaluation questions?

4. One objective of a community program to prevent head injuries is to increase the use of helmets to at least 50% of child and adult bicyclists. What is an impact evaluation question for this objective?

A
C
T *Two*

ANSWERING THE QUESTION

Scene 1: ▶ *Designing the Evaluation*

Once the evaluation questions are defined and Act I comes to a close, the evaluation process enters Act II of the play, where the evaluator applies research methods to obtain an accurate answer for each question. The application of research methods is a *process* that has two basic steps, or scenes: "Scene 1: Designing the Evaluation" and "Scene 2: Planning and Conducting the Evaluation."

In Scene 1, research methods are applied to develop a strategy, or design, for collecting and analyzing data to answer each impact and process question about the program. In general, several designs can be used to answer any given impact or process question; however, some designs yield more accurate answers than others. The evaluator's goal is to choose a design that offers the most accurate answers, within the logistical, budget, and other constraints of the evaluation. In Chapter 4, evaluation designs for determining a program's impacts are described. Chapter 5 extends this material and presents an overview of the cost-effectiveness evaluation of health programs. Scene I concludes with a review of designs for evaluating a program's implementation in Chapter 6.

Once the evaluation design is completed, it becomes a "blueprint" for planning and conducting the evaluation in Scene II. In Chapter 7, methods are described for selecting the population and drawing the sample, which includes the calculation of sample size requirements. Chapter 8 presents methods for measuring program outcomes and implementation, as well as a review of common approaches of collecting data in health program evaluations. Act II of the evaluation process closes with Chapter 9, which examines key issues in organizing and conducting data analyses.

CHAPTER 4

Evaluation of Program Impacts

This chapter explains how to design an evaluation of a health program's impacts. The chapter begins with a discussion of causal inference and its implications for obtaining accurate answers to impact questions. Next, alternative evaluation designs and their relative strengths and weaknesses are reviewed. The remaining sections of the chapter address statistical and measurement issues that can affect the accuracy of impact evaluations. The final section summarizes key issues in choosing an impact design and estimating program effects.

CAUSAL INFERENCE AND THE
VALIDITY OF THE ANSWERS

In the Medicare demonstration described in Chapter 3, an intermediate objective of the demonstration is to increase the healthy behaviors of older adults in the intervention group, who receive a package of health promotion and disease prevention services. If the intervention works as intended, it will *cause* adults who do not perform a healthy behavior, such as regular exercise, to increase their exercise between baseline and follow-up, as shown by Arrow A in Figure 4.1 (Lipsey 1997). Other outcomes are also possible. Older adults who already exercise regularly may continue to do so (Arrow B), or they may stop exercising regularly (Arrow C). Alternatively, the intervention may not work; adults who do not exercise regularly at baseline may exhibit the same behavior at follow-up (Arrow D). In short, older adults may *change* their behavior, as shown by Arrows A and C, or they may *not change* their behavior, as shown by

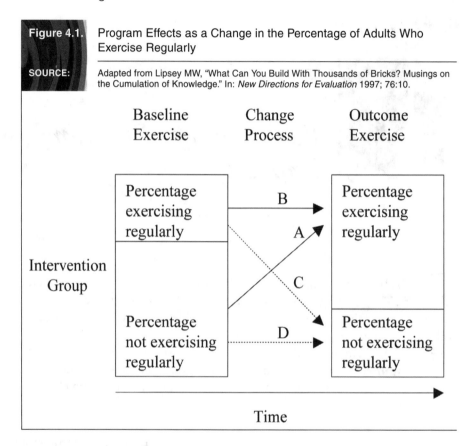

Figure 4.1. Program Effects as a Change in the Percentage of Adults Who Exercise Regularly

SOURCE: Adapted from Lipsey MW, "What Can You Build With Thousands of Bricks? Musings on the Cumulation of Knowledge." In: *New Directions for Evaluation* 1997; 76:10.

Arrows B and D. If the program works as intended, we expect that the program will *cause* adults who do not exercise at baseline to exercise more, which will increase the percentage of older adults who exercise regularly at follow-up (Arrow A).

Causality is the central issue in all impact evaluations. When an impact question is asked, such as "Did the program increase regular exercise among older adults?", we want to know whether any observed changes in exercise behavior are caused by the program rather than by other factors. The ability to make accurate causal inferences about a program's impacts is known as *internal validity* and is an essential requirement of any impact evaluation.

For an impact evaluation to have internal validity, five requirements of causal inference must be satisfied (Blalock 1964; Cook and Campbell 1979; Green and Lewis 1986):

i.v ability to make *causal inf. - DV*

1. A theoretical, conceptual, or practical basis for the expected relationship exists, as defined by the program's theory (see Chapter 3).
2. The program precedes the outcome in time.
3. Other explanations are ruled out.
4. A statistically significant association exists between the program and the outcome (the outcome is not due to chance).
5. Outcome measures are reliable and valid.

The first and second requirements can be satisfied in most impact evaluations. The theoretical, conceptual, or practical rationale for why the program might cause expected changes is specified in the program's theory in Act I of the evaluation process (see Chapter 2). For the second requirement, the implementation of a program occurs before outcomes are observed in most cases, creating a basis for "if X, then Y" causal reasoning.

The remaining three requirements may or may not be satisfied for various reasons, and each of these reasons is called a "threat" to internal validity. To satisfy the third requirement, an impact evaluation must be designed in such a way that other competing explanations for observed outcomes are ruled out. To accomplish this objective, different approaches, or *designs*, for conducting impact evaluations can be applied. They can be classified into three types: (a) *experimental*, (b) *quasi-experimental*, and (c) *pre-experimental*. In general, experimental designs rule out more threats to internal validity than quasi-experimental designs, and quasi-experimental designs rule out more threats than pre-experimental designs, as shown in the "internal validity continuum" in Figure 4.2. In designing an impact evaluation, the goal is to pick a design as far up the continuum as possible that can be applied feasibly to the health program. Because no impact design can rule out all threats, however, *design threats* to internal validity exist in virtually all impact evaluations.

For the fourth requirement of causal inference, threats to *statistical conclusion validity* may exist (Cook and Campbell 1979). Impact evaluations inevitably require the use of statistics, and most statistical procedures have requirements that must be satisfied to draw valid inferences about whether an association exists between the program and observed outcomes. If the requirements are not satisfied, it may be impossible to detect an association between the program and its outcomes, if an association in fact exists.

Making causal inferences also requires reliable and accurate, or valid, measures of program outcomes. If the program's outcome measures are not reliable and valid, *measurement threats* to internal validity also may exist.

| Figure 4.2. | Internal Validity Continuum Showing the Three Types of Impact Evaluation Designs and Their Relative Internal Validity |

LOW   HIGH
INTERNAL   INTERNAL
VALIDITY   VALIDITY

Pre-Experimental   Quasi-Experimental   Experimental
    Designs   Designs   Designs

Up to this point, the focus has been on threats to internal validity, or the ability to make causal inferences about a program's effects. After an impact evaluation of a health program is conducted and results are obtained, a common question is whether the results can be generalized to other settings, which is known as the *external validity* of the results. Internal validity is more important than external validity because impact results cannot be generalized to other settings without first knowing whether the results are due to the program or to other factors.

In summary, three basic types of designs exist for conducting impact evaluations: experimental, quasi-experimental, and pre-experimental. In the sections that follow, the impact designs in each type are reviewed, along with their respective threats to internal and external validity. Next, threats to statistical conclusion and measurement validity are examined. The chapter ends with a discussion of the insights that can be gained from meta-analyses of impact evaluations of health programs.

PRE-EXPERIMENTAL DESIGNS

One-Group Posttest-Only Design

Suppose that you are an administrator of a health maintenance organization (HMO) that provides medical care to more than 300,000 members. The HMO receives a monthly payment for each member, regardless of whether members are sick or healthy. Sick members generally have higher utilization and costs than healthy members and therefore pose greater financial risks for the HMO. You notice that chronically disabled adults over age 65 have health costs seven times as high as those of healthy adults (Pardes et al. 1999), and you and your colleagues decide to launch a pilot health promotion program customized for older adults with chronic illness and higher use of physician services. The HMO assumes that the program will increase the health knowledge and healthy life-styles of older adults, which will slow the decline in health status and depend-ence with aging, resulting in lower utilization and costs in the long run for this population group. To increase the likelihood of success, the pilot program is de-signed for older adults with 10 or more visits to a primary care physician in the previous year. The pilot program is implemented in one of the HMO's clinics, where older adults attend a 2-hour class once a week for 4 weeks.

You receive a report 8 months later describing the program and whether it had actually changed the health knowledge and lifestyles of older adults. To an-swer this question, the impact evaluation asked each adult to complete a mail questionnaire about his or her health knowledge and behaviors 6 months after the program started. More than 80% of the adults completed and returned the questionnaire. Based on the findings, the report indicates that health knowledge and healthy behaviors are relatively high and recommends that the program be expanded to other clinics.

The pre-experimental design for this impact study is known as a *one-group posttest-only design* and is diagramed as follows (Campbell and Stanley 1963; Cook and Campbell 1979; Rog 1994; Shortell and Richardson 1978):

$$X\ O_1$$

where X represents the program and O_1 is the observation of patient knowl-edge, which in this case is the questionnaire. On the basis of your knowledge of impact evaluation, you question the validity of the report's findings because the design has two important threats to internal validity: history and maturation.

History Threats

The positive findings may be due to other events or the experiences of adults occurring between the program and the 6-month follow-up. For example, pro-gram participants may have gained health knowledge from magazine and news-paper articles, television shows, or other mass media communications about health topics. Alternatively, because they visit the doctor often, their health knowledge may have changed through the experience of receiving medical care itself, such as through information provided by their physicians or nurses. His-tory threats are discrete events *external* to subjects occurring between the begin-ning and end of a program that may also explain observed outcomes.

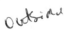

Maturation Threats

The results also may be caused by mental or physical changes occurring *within* the program participants themselves. Participants likely have poor health, and over time they may gain familiarity with and knowledge about their illnesses and disabilities and ways to prevent or manage them, which may also explain observed levels of health knowledge at the 6-month follow-up. Alternatively, participants may experience boredom with the program, which may also account for observed outcomes. In general, the longer the time interval between the start and end of a program, the greater is the maturation threat to internal validity. For example, if the questionnaire follow-up was conducted 2 years after the program, health knowledge may have increased simply because the participants aged 2 years. This is particularly true for health programs targeting children, who are growing and developing both physically and mentally. These internal changes, rather than the program, may explain results. In summary, maturation threats are events or processes occurring *inside* the person with the passage of time, while history refers to events happening *outside* the person, and they may either singly or jointly account for observed outcomes.

One-Group Pretest-Posttest Design

In response to these problems, you consider alternative designs for evaluating the impact of the program. One approach is to measure the patients' knowledge of health care *before* and *after* the program. This approach is called a *one-group pretest-posttest design* and is diagrammed as follows (Campbell and Stanley 1963; Cook and Campbell 1979; Rog 1994; Shortell and Richardson 1978):

$$O_1 \; X \; O_2$$

With this design you can measure the change (increase or decrease, if any) in health knowledge and behavior before and after the program. You also realize, however, that the history and maturation threats also apply to this design, plus some new threats to internal validity, which are described below.

Testing Threats

If a change in health knowledge or behavior is observed, the change may be due not to the program itself but simply to giving patients a test—in this case, a questionnaire assessing their knowledge of care—*before* the program. The questionnaire, or "pretest," may have conveyed knowledge to patients, resulting in higher scores at the 6-month follow-up, or "posttest," regardless of whether the program worked or not. Testing effects may either overstate the true effects of the program, as in this example, or understate the program's effects. In some contexts, the administration of a pretest may create anxiety, lowering performance on the posttest and thereby underestimating the program's true effect.

Instrumentation Threats

At the pretest, let's suppose that program participants were asked 10 knowledge questions. After examining the pretest scores, you discover that all adults answered one of the questions correctly. For the posttest, you decide to revise this item to make it more difficult to answer. Because of this revision, observed changes between the pretest and posttest may be due to changes in the questionnaire, or "instrument," or how it was administered to patients, rather than the program itself. In short, to avoid instrumentation threats, the content and administration of the pretest and posttest instruments must be *identical*. Instrumentation threats exist if questions are asked differently in the pretest and posttest, the interviewers are not the same between tests, or the mode of data collection (personal interview, telephone interview, self-administered questionnaire) changes between the pretest and posttest.

Regression Threats

When the program is announced, more people may want to enroll in the classes than you have room for. You decide to target the class at older adults with relatively little health knowledge. You ask all program applicants to complete the pretest questionnaire, and you enroll those adults with the lowest knowledge scores (other adults are put on a waiting list). When you administer the posttest, the average posttest scores are much higher. Is the increase in health knowledge due to the program? Probably not, for when participants are selected because they have extremely low pretest scores, their posttest scores will tend to shift *upward* toward the mean score for all older adults in the clinic, regardless of whether the program worked or not. Similarly, if participants are selected because they have extremely high levels of knowledge, their posttest scores will naturally regress *downward* toward the population mean.

This regression threat to internal validity exists only when people are enrolled into a program based on their extreme pretest scores. If a program does not select people based on their extreme pretest scores, the regression threat does not apply to the program.

TABLE 4.1   Regression Between Pretest and Posttest Scores

Pretest Scores	Posttest Scores							Mean Posttest
	7	8	9	10	11	12	13	
13				1	1	1	1	11.5
12			1	1	2	1	1	11.0
11		1	2	3	3	2	1	10.5
10	1	1	3	4	3	1	1	10.0
9	1	2	3	3	2	1		9.5
8	1	1	2	1	1			9.0
7	1	1	1	1				8.5
Mean Pretest	8.5	9.0	9.5	10.0	10.5	11.0	11.5	

SOURCE: Adapted from Campbell, Donald T., and Julian C. Stanley, *Experimental and Quasi-Experimental Designs for Research*, p. 10. Copyright © 1963 by Houghton Mifflin Company. Used with permission.

The regression threat is illustrated in Table 4.1, which presents hypothetical pretest and posttest scores for an education program (Campbell and Stanley 1963; Shortell and Richardson 1978). Pretest scores are the rows of the matrix and range between 7 and 13. Posttest scores are the columns of the matrix and also range between 7 and 13. The bottom row consists of four persons who had the lowest pretest score of 7. Only one of the four persons also had a 7 posttest score; the other 3 persons had higher posttest scores of 8, 9, and 10.

The posttest scores may be higher for any number of reasons. For example, at the pretest the four persons may not have slept well the night before the test, or they may not have understood the questions, or they may have been distracted by family illness, and so forth. At the posttest, the scores are higher, averaging 8.5, and more accurately reflect the persons' knowledge because, other things equal, they would likely have slept well the night before, experience gained from the pretest would have reduced the number of misunderstood questions, and family illnesses may have improved. Put another way, the likelihood of the four persons with the lowest score on the pretest also scoring *exactly* the same score on the posttest is relatively small; therefore, the pretest and posttest scores of the four persons will be less than perfectly correlated (1.0). A similar pattern also exists for the four persons with the highest pretest score (13), which regress downward to 10, 11, and 12. For all persons in Table 4.1, the correlation between the pretest and posttest scores is .50, with no change in the group mean (10.0) or variance.

Just how much extreme pretest scores regress toward the population mean depends on two factors: (a) the test-retest reliability of the measure and (b) the difference between the mean of the deliberately selected group with extreme pretest scores and the mean of the population from which the group was chosen. Test-retest reliability is the correlation between the scores of a test or questionnaire administered at two different but relatively close points in time, such as a week apart. The higher the test-retest correlation, the more reliable is the measure. In general, the greater the reliability of a measure and the smaller the difference between the means, the less regression there will be (Cook and Campbell 1979).

As a final point, persons may be selected to participate in a program for reasons totally unrelated to their pretest scores. It may still turn out, however, that the persons have either extremely low or high pretest scores. In this case, the pretest extreme scores are less likely to regress toward the mean at the posttest, mainly because a variety of random factors would likely affect the pretest scores. This would not be the case, however, for persons selected *because* of their extreme scores.

Posttest-Only Comparison Group Design

After considering advantages and disadvantages of the pretest-posttest design, you decide to discard the pretest because it eliminates the testing, instrumentation, and regression threats. Instead, you decide to add a *comparison group* composed of older adults with 10 or more physician visits in the past year at a *different* clinic where the program does not exist. This approach is called a *posttest-only comparison group design* and is diagrammed as follows (Campbell and Stanley 1963; Cook and Campbell 1979; Rog 1994; Shortell and Richardson 1978):

$$X\ O_1$$
$$\dotfill$$
$$O_2$$

In this design, a dashed, horizontal line is used to define the group receiving the program and the comparison group. By convention, the group receiving the intervention appears above the line. The X indicates the health promotion program, and O_1 indicates the posttest observation, or measure, of the health knowledge and behavior among participants in the clinic with the program. The comparison group appears below the line and consists of persons with similar characteristics who did not receive the program. In this case, O_2 is the observation or measure of knowledge and behavior among older adults from the clinic without the program. The horizontal line is dashed to indicate that the individuals have not been randomized to the intervention and comparison groups, and, therefore, the two groups were not equivalent at the beginning of the program. Program effects are determined by comparing the health knowledge and behavior in the program group (O_1) with the health knowledge and behavior in the comparison group (O_2). In epidemiology, this design is known as a case-control study and also is referred to as a static group comparison design in the program evaluation literature.

In the posttest-only comparison group design, you can rule out testing, instrumentation, and regression threats because those threats apply to the administration of a pretest, which the design lacks. For the most part, history threats also can be ruled out because any events (such as a newspaper article, a television show, or a new book) disseminating health information that might affect the posttest scores of the intervention group would also affect the comparison group. Thus, any difference between the O_1 and O_2 scores would be attributable to the program because the exposure to such outside, or historical, events was essentially the same between groups. *Intra-session history* is an exception to this case. That is, by virtue of being in the intervention group, the people in the intervention group experienced historical events that the comparison group did not. For example, because the program participants actually meet as a group, they may exchange information about health care above and beyond what the classes provide. In these cases, any difference between the intervention and comparison group may be due to such factors and not exposure to the program.

Selection Threats

If a statistically significant difference exists in the average posttest scores of the intervention and comparison groups, the difference may be due to the program, or it may be due to preexisting differences in the people in the two groups. When the characteristics of the intervention group and the comparison group are significantly different from each other, the different characteristics between the groups, rather than the program itself, may account for the difference in the posttest scores. For example, compared to adults in the comparison clinic, the adults in the intervention clinic may be sicker and therefore have more opportunity, skills, or motivation to learn health information or change their behavior.

Selection formally refers to differences in the composition of the intervention and comparison groups that account for observed outcomes, and it is the major threat to internal validity in the posttest-only comparison group design. Its title underscores the fact that program effects are estimated by *comparing* the intervention group with another, nonequivalent group. The difference in the average posttest scores between the intervention and comparison groups depends on the effect of the program (if any) *and* how similar or different the two groups are. Thus, the choice of a comparison group is a critical decision when using this design. Selection threats can be reduced, but not eliminated, by choosing a comparison group that is similar as possible to the intervention group.

Interactions With Selection

Selection threats may operate jointly with maturation, history, and instrumentation threats to internal validity. The *interaction of selection and maturation* may occur, for example, if the persons in the intervention group are sicker than those in the comparison group, which by itself is a selection threat to internal validity. If the health of the persons in the intervention group began or continued to decline (a case of maturation), they may learn more about health care because of their increased interest and awareness of their declining health, and not because of the program itself.

Similarly, the *interaction of selection and history* occurs when the intervention and comparison groups have different characteristics, and because of these differences the two groups experience historical events in different ways. For example, patients in the intervention and comparison clinics may come from different cultural groups, a selection threat. Because people from different cultures may interpret historical events differently, observed differences between the clinics may be due to these interpretations rather than to the program itself. Selection and history also may interact when groups come from different settings and, as a consequence, each group experiences a unique local history that might affect program outcomes. For example, the waiting rooms of the intervention and comparison clinics may have racks stocked with health information booklets, but the health topics of the booklets are different between clinics, and therefore, older adults in each clinic are exposed to unique historical events.

The *interaction of selection and instrumentation* may occur when the two groups have different characteristics and consequently have different scores on an instrument with unequal intervals. For example, a variety of scales exists to measure health status. If persons in the intervention group are sicker (a selection effect), they may score at the lower end of the health status scale, while the healthy persons in the comparison group may score at the high end of the scale. The interaction of selection and instrumentation occurs when the health status scale cannot detect any more gains in the healthy group (a "ceiling effect"), or when the scale cannot detect any further decline in the sicker group (a "floor effect").

Attrition

In the health promotion program for older adults, let's suppose that the program begins in March. The comparison group is drawn from another clinic without the program. To reduce selection threats to internal invalidity, each patient in the intervention group is matched with a randomly selected patient in the comparison clinic having the same age and gender (Friedman 1994; MacMahon and Trichopoulus 1996). Six months later, you measure the health knowledge of older adults in each group (that is, the posttest scores in the study design) by conducting a telephone interview of each person. In the course of conducting the interviews, you discover that 1% of the adults in the intervention group have died, while 10% of the adults in the comparison group have died. With the loss of the sickest adults in the comparison group, the remaining adults in the comparison group are healthier than the remaining adults in the intervention group. Because sicker adults generally have more experience with disease and health care, the results show that average knowledge scores are higher in the intervention group than in the comparison group. In this case, the higher scores in the intervention group are due to attrition rather than to the program itself.

Formally stated, attrition threats occur when different kinds of persons drop out of the two groups having initial similar characteristics. The differential dropout rates change the composition of the groups, thereby introducing a selection threat to internal validity (because the persons in the two groups are no longer similar).

In summary, the three pre-experimental designs are subject to ten different threats to internal validity, which are defined in Table 4.2.

TABLE 4.2   Summary of Threats to Internal Validity in Pre-Experimental Impact
Designs

1. *History:* Discrete events external to the subjects
2. *Maturation:* Events occurring within subjects as a systematic function of time
3. *Testing:* Providing a pretest that may affect subjects in either a positive or a negative fashion such as to influence results
4. *Instrumentation:* Changes in the measuring instrument or those administering the measuring instrument that might cause changes in the program results
5. *Regression artifacts:* Where subjects have been selected on the basis of their extreme scores, program results will be affected by the fact that these extreme scores will have naturally regressed toward the mean
6. *Selection:* Differences in the composition of subjects making up the intervention and comparison groups
7. *Attrition:* Differential dropout of subjects between the intervention and comparison group
8. *Selection-maturation interaction:* Differences in maturation effects due to selection differences in the composition of subjects making up the intervention and comparison groups
9. *Selection-history interaction:* Differences in exposure to or interpretation of historical events due to selection differences in the composition of subjects making up the intervention and comparison groups
10. *Selection-instrumentation interaction:* Differences in instrument scores that are due to selection differences in the composition of subjects making up the intervention and comparison groups.

SOURCE: Adapted from Shortell SM, Richardson WC. *Health Program Evaluation.* St. Louis, MO: Mosby Company; 1978:44.

External Validity

A common question with pre-experimental and other types of impact designs is whether the results of the impact evaluation can be applied, or generalized, to other populations, settings, or time periods, which is also referred to as the *external validity* of the results. If threats to internal validity exist, external validity also is threatened. If we assume that most threats to internal validity can be ruled out, five threats to external validity still may undermine the generalizability of the findings:

1. Interaction of selection and treatment,
2. Interaction of testing and treatment,

3. Interaction of setting and treatment (also known as situation or "reactive" effects),

4. Interaction of history and treatment, and

5. Multiple treatment effects.

Selection-treatment interaction threats pose the following question: Do the results of an impact evaluation also apply to other groups with different characteristics? In the example for the posttest-only comparison group design, the impact of the health promotion program based on the findings from one clinic may not be generalizable to other clinics that have older adult populations with different characteristics. This problem can be reduced by expanding the program and sampling different clinics with different populations, and then conducting the impact evaluation on a larger scale across these heterogeneous settings. Selection-treatment interaction also is a problem in evaluations like "A Healthy Future," in which 5,012 Medicare enrollees were invited to participate in the program but only about half consented to do so. In such cases, the findings are applicable only to the volunteers and may not apply to the larger population from which they were sampled, and clearly not to other Medicare enrollees across the nation. The threat applies to all three pre-experimental designs.

Testing-treatment interaction threats pose the following question: Can the results of an impact evaluation with a pretest be obtained when the program is implemented without a pretest? If a program has beneficial effects, those results may be generalizable to other contexts only when a pretest also is administered. This threat is relevant when the administration of a pretest influences the behavior of participants in the program that follows. Thus, if the same program is repeated without the pretest and smaller benefits are obtained, any drop in performance may reflect not program failure but rather the absence of the pretest. This threat applies only to the design with a pretest, the pretest-posttest design.

Setting and treatment interaction threats pose the following question: Can the results of an impact evaluation obtained in one setting be generalized to other settings? For example, the results of the health promotion program implemented in an HMO may not be generalizable to non-HMO settings. Setting-treatment interactions also are a threat when specific features of the program itself are not replicated in other settings, leading to different results. For example, a health promotion program may be highly effective because the instructor has a charismatic, engaging personality. If the same program is administered by a person without those qualities, identical program effects may not be observed. Similarly, if persons are aware they are participating in an experiment, they may be more (or less) motivated to perform well (the "Hawthorne effect"), thereby producing outcomes that are higher or lower than expected without such an awareness. Alternatively, a new program may generate enthusiasm among participants in the treatment group, producing big program effects. The program's generalizability, however, may be limited to settings where it is being newly introduced. The threat applies to all three designs.

History-treatment interaction threats pose the following question: Can the results obtained today be generalized to past or future periods? Short-term historical threats may occur when a program is implemented, by chance, on the same day that a prominent event also occurs. For example, a high school program to prevent youth violence may be launched, by coincidence, on the same day that gunshots are fired in another, nearby high school. The effects of the violence prevention program may be contingent on the occurrence of violence in the youth community on the same day and therefore may not be generalizable to periods when such events do not occur. Long-term historical threats may occur, for example, when an effective program to reduce teenage pregnancy developed in the 1970s is implemented in the 1990s. Because historical events concerning birth control may be different between the two decades, the 1970s findings may not be generalizable to the later period. This threat applies to all three pre-experimental designs.

Multiple treatment threats pose the following question: If the program is just one of several programs in a setting, can the impact results for that program be generalized to other settings that do not have the other programs? Many health care organizations have implemented multiple programs to achieve diverse goals. It is becoming more and more common for the same people to be in the treatment group of more than one program. When this occurs, the beneficial effects of one program may be contingent on the treatment group's participation in other health programs. In this context, program effects may be generalizable only to those settings where the treatment group also participates in other, identical programs. This threat applies to all designs.

SUMMARY

Pre-experimental designs consist of the one-group posttest-only design, the pretest-posttest design, and the posttest-only comparison group design. At least two threats to internal validity apply to each design, as shown in Table 4.3. Because the one-group posttest-only design has serious threats to internal validity, it is rarely used to evaluate the impacts of health programs. In contrast, the pretest-posttest design and the posttest-only comparison group design are used more frequently to evaluate the impacts of health programs (for example, see

TABLE 4.3   Summary of Potential Threats to Validity for Three Pre-Experimental Designs[a]

	Internal								External			
	History	Maturation	Testing	Instrumentation	Regression	Selection	Attrition	Interaction of selection and maturation, etc.	Interaction of testing and X	Interaction of selection and X	Interaction of setting/history and X	Multiple-X interference
1. One-group posttest-only X O_1	−	−	+	+	+	+	+	−	+	−	?	?
2. One-group pretest-posttest O_1 X O_2	−	−	−	−	−	+	+	−	−	−	?	?
3. Posttest-only comparison group X O_1 ――― O_2	+	+	+	+	+	−	−	−	+	−	?	?

SOURCE: Adapted from Campbell, Donald T., and Julian C. Stanley, *Experimental and Quasi-Experimental Designs for Research*, p. 8. Copyright © 1963 by Houghton Mifflin Company. Used with permission.

a. The "+" indicates the design controls for a potential threat to internal validity, a "−" indicates a definite weakness, and a "?" indicates a possible source of concern. The "X" indicates the program.

Griffin et al. 1999; Hannan et al. 1994; Krieger et al. 1992; Meischke et al. 1999; Rogers et al. 1991). Both prospective and retrospective evaluations of program impacts can be conducted using the posttest-only comparison group design. Some retrospective program evaluations, however, cannot be conducted using the pretest-posttest design, such as when the pretest is a questionnaire that must be completed by individuals before the program starts. The external validity threats generally apply to all the pre-experimental designs, as well as to all the other designs on the internal validity continuum in Figure 4.2, which are addressed in the next sections.

EXPERIMENTAL DESIGNS

Pretest-Posttest Control Group Design

Even though you have carefully matched older adults in the intervention and comparison groups in the posttest-only comparison group design, selection threats to internal validity may still exist (Grossman and Tierney 1993). To eliminate selection threats, you decide to randomly allocate older adults to the intervention and control groups. Randomization is chosen because it increases the likelihood that intervention and control groups are alike before the intervention group is exposed to the program, which allows you to rule out alternative explanations for program results. Randomization is important particularly when program effects are expected to be small, which may be the case for your health promotion program for older adults (Shortell and Richardson 1978).

The next time the health promotion class is offered, you invite older adults with 10 or more physician visits in the past year at another HMO clinic to attend the program. Half consent to do so, and you randomly allocate half of the volunteers to the intervention group and half to the control group. This "true" experimental design is known as a *pretest-posttest control group design* and is diagramed as follows (Campbell and Stanley 1963):

$$R \; O_1 \; X \; O_2$$
$$R \; O_3 \; \quad O_4$$

The two Rs indicate that older adults are randomized to the intervention and control groups. The absence of a dashed line indicates the bottom group is a "true" control group due to randomization. The X indicates the administration of the program to the intervention group, and O_1 and O_2 are the pretest and posttest observations for the intervention group. The O_3 and O_4 indicate the pretest and posttest observations for the control group. Program effects are estimated by calculating the average difference between the pretest and posttest scores in the intervention group $(O_2 - O_1)$, or "gain score," and the average difference between the scores for the control group $(O_4 - O_3)$. If the program worked, the average gain scores for the intervention group should be significantly greater than the average gain scores in the control group. For example, in the health promotion program for older adults, we would expect that adults in the intervention group would have greater gains in health knowledge and the performance of healthy behaviors than the adults in the control group.

Located at the opposite end of the internal validity continuum in Figure 4.2, randomized experimental designs generally eliminate most threats to internal validity, except attrition. *History threats* are controlled because external events that affect the intervention group also affect the control group. Intra-session history, however, remains a possible threat.

Maturation threats are eliminated through randomization, which increases the likelihood that events occurring within people (if any) are similar between the two groups.

Testing threats are controlled because each group is exposed to the same test. If the pretest affected people's behavior, it would do so in both groups in similar ways, given randomization.

Instrumentation threats are controlled *if* the pretests and posttests are identical, and if the mode of data collection is the same for the pretest and posttest. If interviewers are used to collect the pretest and posttest measures, the interviewers should have no knowledge of whether a person is in the intervention or control group. The interviewer who collected the pretest observations from a group of older adults should also collect the posttest measures from those adults.

Regression threats are controlled through randomization. If regression to the mean occurs, randomization increases the likelihood that it will be similar in the intervention and control groups; therefore, any differences between the intervention and control groups will be due to the program rather than to regression artifacts.

Selection threats are controlled through randomization, which increases the likelihood that the intervention and control groups are similar at the beginning of the program. Many investigators compare the average values of the O_1 and O_3 pretest scores to verify that no statistically significant differences exist between the two groups (that is, that randomization "worked").

Attrition threats are never ruled out in any experimental design. Put another way, randomization does not eliminate all threats to internal validity, and therefore, no experimental design is at the maximum "high" endpoint of the internal validity continuum in Figure 4.2. With a control group and pretest and posttest observations, however, the extent of differential attrition between the intervention groups can be assessed empirically.

Interaction threats also are controlled, provided that randomization has worked and the two groups are equivalent.

Other threats also may exist in experimental designs. Randomization is a very useful tool for increasing internal validity, or the ability of the evaluator to conclude whether observed differences between the intervention and control groups are actually due to the program versus other causes. Randomization, however, does not eliminate all threats to internal validity. In the course of implementing programs in the field, the following five threats may arise in randomized designs or nonrandomized designs with a control or comparison group, respectively (Cook and Campbell 1979).

> *Diffusion or imitation of the program:* In all designs with a control or comparison group, diffusion or imitation of the program occurs when people in the intervention group communicate with people in the control group. For example, because the older adults in the health promotion program are high users of health services, there is a possibility that adults in the intervention group may share program information with people in the control group whom they happen to meet in the waiting room of the clinic. When this "contamination" problem occurs, there are no planned differences between the intervention and control group, invalidating the entire evaluation.
>
> *Compensatory equalization of treatments:* This is another source of contamination caused by program administrators. When an intervention provides health services that are highly desirable, and the people in the intervention and control groups would both benefit from receiving them, program administrators may become uncomfortable with the inequality that emerges from withholding the services from the control group. To correct the inequality, program administrators may begin offering the program to people in the control group, eliminating the planned contrast between the two groups.
>
> *Compensatory rivalry by people receiving less desirable treatments:* Participation in programs with randomization requires the consent of the participants. If a program is providing desirable services to the intervention group, people in the control group usually are aware that they are receiv-

ing less desirable services. In response to the inequality, social competition between groups may occur, with the "underdog" control group motivated to outperform the "better-off" intervention group, reducing or reversing the expected difference between the groups. Compensatory rivalry is more likely to occur when natural groups (such as classrooms, clinics, or divisions of a health department) are assigned to the intervention and control groups, or when the control group will be worse off if the program works. For example, suppose that a public health department contracts with private clinics to immunize children, where payment is based on the number of immunizations. If clinics are randomized into a program to boost immunization rates, control clinics may perceive the program as a threat to their future performance and revenue, which might undermine future contracts with the health department. The control clinics therefore work harder to outperform the competition. This "John Henry effect" may lead to smaller differences between intervention and control groups.

Resentful demoralization of respondents receiving less desirable treatments: If highly desirable services are withheld from people in the control group, they may become resentful or demoralized about their deprivation. In response, they may become less motivated, become angry, or become less productive or cooperative. These responses would lead to greater differences between the intervention and control groups, and part of the difference would not be due to the program.

Ambiguity about the direction of causal inference: Suppose that a strong, positive correlation between health status and physician visits is found in the treatment group of a posttest-only comparison group design. Do more physician visits result in better health, or does poor health result in more physician visits? Making causal inferences about the program is difficult when associations are obtained from correlational, cross-section studies. This threat does not apply to designs where the temporal ordering of the program and the pretest and posttest observations are clear.

Posttest-Only Control Group Design

The pretest-posttest control group design is widely used to evaluate the impacts of health programs, including the impact of the Medicare demonstration described in Chapter 3 (Patrick et al. 1999). If this design is used to evaluate the impacts of the health promotion program for older adults, and if the program has beneficial effects, there may be great interest in implementing the program in other settings. The external validity of program effects may be threatened, however, by testing-treatment interactions (that is, the beneficial results may be obtained only when a pretest is administered). To address this concern, the impacts of the program without a pretest can be evaluated using a *posttest-only control group design*, as diagramed below (Campbell and Stanley 1963; Shortell and Richardson 1978). The design

Post test Only Control Group Design

$$R \; X \; O_1$$

$$R \quad O_2$$

is similar to the posttest-only *comparison* group design, but the addition of randomization rules out most threats to internal validity, except attrition. If a statistically significant difference exists between the average posttest score of the intervention group (O_1) and the average posttest score of the control group (O_2), the difference between the posttest scores of the two groups can be attributed to the program. This conclusion, however, depends greatly on the assumption that randomization has in fact produced equivalent intervention and control groups at the start of the study. Because pretest observations of key outcome measures do not exist in most cases, this assumption typically cannot be verified. The exception occurs when a pretest "proxy" measure exists that is correlated strongly with the outcome measure. For example, the aim of a program may be to increase health status among adults, measured at the posttest by a self-administered questionnaire. *If* the adults' average health status is correlated highly with average physician visits, and *if* an information system contains pretest observations of physician visits for adults in the intervention and control groups, the equivalence of the two groups may be assessed indirectly by comparing their average number of annual physician visits before the program was implemented.

The posttest-only design also is very useful when the goal of the impact evaluation is to compare the *outcomes* of the intervention and control groups, rather than compare the *change* (between the pretest and posttest) in the intervention group with the change in the control group. For example, Martin and her colleagues (1989) used a posttest-only control group design to evaluate the impact of a primary care physician gatekeeper on health service utilization. Individuals were randomized to identical health plans, one with a gatekeeper and one without, and average utilization and charges for health services over the subsequent 12 months were compared between the gatekeeper and non-gatekeeper groups.

Solomon Four-Group Design

Rather than simply using the posttest-only design, impact evaluations may want to measure the testing-treatment interaction threat to external validity. Named after its originator, the *Solomon four-group design* may be used for this purpose and is diagramed below (Campbell and Stanley 1963; Shortell and Richardson 1978):

$$R \; O_1 \; X \; O_2$$

$$R \; O_3 \quad O_4$$

$$R \quad X \; O_5$$

$$R \quad\quad O_6$$

The design combines the pretest-posttest control group design (top two rows) with the posttest-only control group design (bottom two rows). With four randomized groups, testing-interaction threats can be assessed explicitly. If $O_2 - O_1 > O_4 - O_3$, the program has beneficial effects, but the results may not be generalizable without the pretest. If $O_5 > O_6$, however, testing-treatment interaction threats to external validity can be ruled out. The magnitude of the testing-treatment interaction can be measured explicitly in two steps: (a) calculate the difference in outcomes between the control group with the pretest and the group without the pretest ($O_4 - O_6$), and the difference in outcomes between the intervention groups with and without the pretest ($O_2 - O_5$), then (b) statistically test whether these differences are similar ($O_4 - O_6 = O_2 - O_5$). If they are significantly different from each other, testing-treatment interaction threats exist, measured by the magnitude of the inequality between the two difference scores (Shortell and Richardson 1978). The major disadvantage of the Solomon four-group design is the additional costs and logistics associated with having four rather than two groups. For this reason, the design rarely is used to evaluate the impacts of health programs.

External Validity

None of the experimental designs rules out threats to external validity (Campbell and Stanley 1963). Two exceptions exist. Because the posttest-only control group design lacks a pretest, testing-treatment interaction threats are eliminated in the design. Similarly, because the Solomon four-group design examines impacts with and without a pretest, testing-treatment interaction threats to external validity also are controlled by this design.

When to Randomize

In randomized impact designs, a key decision is *when* to randomize cases to the intervention and control groups. One approach is to randomly assign individuals to the intervention and control groups before the evaluator asks them to participate in the evaluation. This approach has an important disadvantage. Because participation is voluntary, some people may not consent to participate in the evaluation. When this happens, randomization is disrupted, and the treatment and control groups may no longer be equivalent.

An alternative approach is to invite individuals to participate in the evaluation, then randomize only those individuals who consent to participate. The advantage of this approach is that randomization (if it works) yields equivalent groups of participants at baseline. The disadvantage of this approach is that the findings of the impact evaluation are generalizable only to cases who consent to randomization, and not to the original sample.

Although the random assignment of cases to treatment and control groups might appear straightforward, sometimes programs do not implement the random assignment successfully in the field. Conner (1977) and Cook and Campbell (1979) describe major obstacles to random assignment in field settings and methods for overcoming them.

QUASI-EXPERIMENTAL DESIGNS

Quasi-experimental designs are in the middle of the internal validity continuum in Figure 4.2. They are "quasi"-experimental designs because they do not randomize cases to intervention and control groups, and therefore generally have less internal validity than experimental designs. Nevertheless, quasi-experimental designs have features that rule out many threats to internal validity, approximating the advantages of true experimental designs and surpassing pre-experimental designs in their ability to draw causal inferences about program effects. Quasi-experimental designs are used frequently to evaluate the impacts of health programs for several reasons:

▶ Randomization of cases to intervention and control groups is impossible because of logistical constraints.

▶ Ethical, political, or legal issues prohibit randomization.

▶ No viable control group is available.

▶ Primary data cannot be collected at the pretest and posttest.

▶ Resources are inadequate to conduct a randomized design.

▶ A randomized design is implemented but fails during program implementation, such as when the control group also is exposed to the intervention.

Table 4.4 presents common quasi-experimental designs and their threats to internal and external validity. A quick inspection of Table 4.4 indicates that the designs vary in their ability to rule out threats to internal validity; no single design is necessarily superior for an impact evaluation. In addition, the designs generally do not control for most threats to external validity, and therefore generalizability is always a concern. A review of each design in the table follows.

Single Time Series Design

Suppose you wanted to evaluate the impacts of a local health department program to increase immunization rates for newborns in low-income families covered by Medicaid health insurance. Although a pretest-posttest design could be used to estimate program effects, you are concerned that with this design observed differences in immunization rates could be due to history threats (exposure to information about preventive services through the mass media or visits with pediatricians and nurses) or maturation threats (change in the fertility rates of Medicaid women). To reduce these threats to internal validity, you choose a single time series design, an extension of the pretest-posttest design where *multiple* observations are performed *before* and *after* the program, as shown in Figure 4.3 (Cook and Campbell 1979; Marcantonio and Cook 1994; Reichardt and Mark 1998; Shortell and Richardson 1978). The horizontal line represents time, where the O_1, O_2, and O_3 are annual immunization rates in the 3 years before the program was implemented, X indicates the introduction of the program, and O_4, O_5, and O_6 represent annual immunization rates in the

TABLE 4.4   Summary of Potential Threats to Validity for Six Quasi-Experimental Designs[a]

	Internal								External			
	History	Maturation	Testing	Instrumentation	Regression	Selection	Attrition	Interaction of selection and maturation, etc.	Interaction of testing and X	Interaction of selection and X	Interaction of setting/ history and X	Multiple-X interference
1. Single time series $O_1\ O_2\ O_3\ X\ O_4\ \ O_5\ \ O_6$	−	+	+	?	+	+	?	+	−	?	?	?
2. Multiple time series $O_1\ O_2\ O_3\ X\ O_4\ \ O_5\ \ O_6$ $O_7\ O_8\ O_9\ \ \ \ O_{10}\ O_{11}\ O_{12}$	+	+	+	+	+	?	?	+	−	−	?	?
3. Repeated treatment design $O_1\ O_2\ X\ O_3\ O_4{-}X\ O_5\ O_6\ X\ O_7\ O_8{-}X\ O_9O_{10}$	+	+	+	?	+	+	?	+	−	?	−	?
4. Nonequivalent comparison group design $O_1\ X\ O_2$ $O_3\ \ \ \ O_4$	+	+	+	+	?	?	?	−	−	?	?	?
5. Institutional cycle design $X\ O_1$ $\ \ O_2\ X\ O_3$ $\ \ \ \ \ \ \ \ \ O_4$	+	−	+	+	−	?	?	−	+	?	?	?
6. Regression discontinuity design	+	+	+	?	+	+	?	+	+	−	?	?

SOURCE: Adapted from Campbell, Donald T., and Julian C. Stanley, *Experimental and Quasi-Experimental Designs for Research*, pp. 40, 56. Copyright © 1963 by Houghton Mifflin Company. Used with permission.

a. The "+" indicates the design controls for a potential threat to internal validity, a "−" indicates a definite weakness, and a "?" indicates a possible source of concern. The "X" indicates the program.

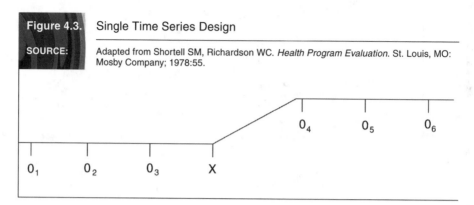

Figure 4.3. Single Time Series Design

SOURCE: Adapted from Shortell SM, Richardson WC. *Health Program Evaluation*. St. Louis, MO: Mosby Company; 1978:55.

3 years after the program began. To be convinced that the program caused an increase in immunization rates, you expect to see an abrupt change in the rates before and after the program was implemented (between O_3 and O_4). The general form of the single time series design is presented below (Campbell and Stanley 1963; Shortell and Richardson 1978):

$$O_1 \; O_2 \; O_3 \; X \; O_4 \; O_5 \; O_6$$

The single (or "interrupted") time series design controls for more threats to internal validity than the pretest-posttest design. *Maturation* threats are controlled, for if the change in immunization rates between O_3 and O_4 was due to changes in fertility rates, these changes also should be observed between O_1 and O_2 as well as O_2 and O_3.

History threats are controlled partially. For a historical event to be a plausible alternative explanation for the change between O_3 and O_4, the event must be unique and specific to that period and not to the previous periods (O_1, O_2, and O_3). Thus, *if* mass media coverage of child immunizations or other preventive services began at O_1, and *if* the coverage can cause immunization rates to increase, immunization rates also should increase between O_1 and O_2 as well as O_2 and O_3. If media coverage was present at O_1 and rates do not increase in the pre-program period, as shown in Figure 4.3, media coverage may be ruled out as a viable alternative explanation of program effects.

Testing threats are controlled because they tend to diminish over time and because they are unlikely to occur only when the program begins. Put another way, if the change between O_3 and O_4 were due to testing effects, those changes also should be observed between O_1 and O_2 and between O_2 and O_3.

Instrumentation is a threat to internal validity *if* the introduction of the program also is associated with changes in the way observations are defined or recorded. For example, if the age group for calculating the immunization rates was changed at O_3, the increase between O_3 and O_4 may be due to the change in measurement rather than to the program. Similarly, if data are collected by observers or interviewers, the data collectors may experience boredom or fatigue over time, which may alter how they perform their observations. Alternatively, if data collectors are aware of when the program is introduced, they may unconsciously change their recording practices in ways that favor the program.

Regression usually is not a problem because regression toward the mean tends to decline over time. For example, the immunization program may target children with very low immunization rates at O_1. Between O_1 and O_2 and between O_2 and O_3, their immunization rates would regress upward toward the mean before the program starts, providing a benchmark for judging whether changes occurred after the program is implemented.

Selection is not a threat because the design has no control group. *Attrition* is not controlled, but it can be assessed by comparing dropout rates (for example, children leaving the Medicaid program) over time. If the dropout rate between O_3 and O_4 is similar to the dropout rate for other periods, attrition threats may be less of a problem. Even though the dropout rates are similar over time, however, the characteristics of the children in the program may still be changing over time as a result of the attrition. Thus, the design does not eliminate attrition threats.

External validity is threatened mainly by testing-treatment interaction, and the remaining threats also may apply, depending on the presence or absence of setting and multiple treatment effects, as well as the characteristics of cases targeted by the program. If the program is replicated in a variety of settings and populations, and similar results are obtained, the external validity of program effects is increased.

A time series may take the shape illustrated in Figure 4.3, or it may have different patterns, as shown in Figure 4.4 (Reichardt 1992). Patterns A through G illustrate different types of program effects. A program could produce an immediate change in the level and/or slope of the observations (patterns A, B, and C). Alternatively, the program's effects may be delayed (patterns D and E) or temporary (patterns F and G). If a program effect is delayed or temporary, the length of the delay or the timing of the effect *must* be clearly predicted by the program's theory of cause and effect. This is because the longer the delay between the start of the program and the start of the change, the greater the likelihood that historical events may account for them. Abrupt changes provide

Figure 4.4.   Interpretation of Single Time Series Observations

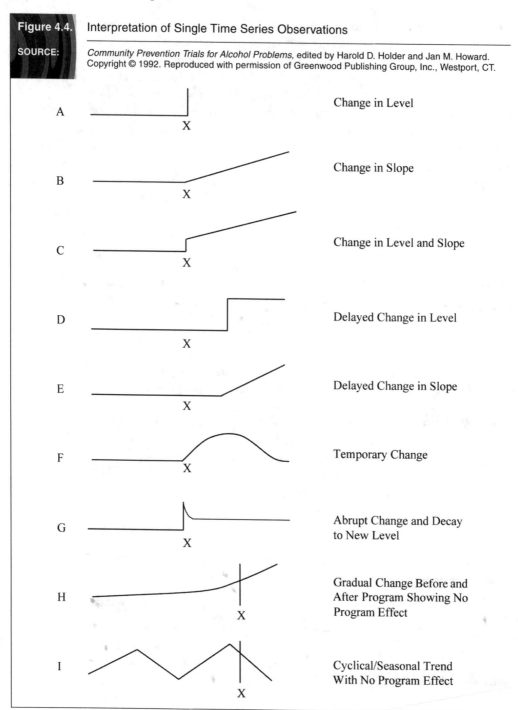

more confidence that a program effect exists, whereas gradual changes may simply reflect trends that would exist even if the program was not implemented, as shown in pattern H. The time series design also is not well suited for evaluating programs that are subject to cyclical or seasonal shifts, as shown in pattern I, where the change between O_4 and O_5 is due to the timing of program implementation and not to the program itself.

Time series designs can be used in prospective and retrospective evaluations of program impacts. Prospective evaluations can pinpoint the exact time when a program starts, which can improve the interpretation of time series observations. The design is well suited for retrospective evaluations where continuous data for previous periods exist for the program's outcome measures. For example, Fleming and Becker (1992) used the design to determine the impact of a motorcycle helmet law on head-related fatalities in Texas by comparing motor vehicle traffic accident reports before and after the law was implemented.

On a final note, researchers also are using the single time series design to make causal inferences about whether deaths following natural disasters are due to the disaster itself or other reasons. For example, Leor and associates (1996) used the design to pinpoint whether the Los Angeles earthquake on January 17, 1994, caused an increase in sudden cardiac deaths on the day of the earthquake. Similarly, Krug and associates (1998) used a single time series design to determine whether natural disasters (such as floods, hurricanes, and earthquakes) caused an increase in suicide rates.

Multiple Time Series Design

To rule out history threats in the single time series evaluation of the immunization program for newborns covered by Medicaid, you decide to add a comparison group composed of newborns covered by Medicaid in an adjacent county where the program does not exist, creating a multiple time series design, which is diagramed below. The dashed line indicates that cases are not randomly assigned to groups.

$$O_1\ O_2\ O_3\ O_4\ X\ O_5\ O_6\ O_7\ O_8$$
$$-----------------------------$$
$$O_9\ O_{10}\ O_{11}\ O_{12}\quad O_{13}\ O_{14}\ O_{15}\ O_{16}$$

Multiple observations are collected before and after the program is launched for both groups. By adding a comparison group, the design controls for history

Figure 4.5a. Trends in Neonatal Mortality in the Intervention (RICP) Counties and the Comparison (non-RICP) Counties, 1964-1984.

SOURCE: Gortmaker SL, Clark CJB, Graven SN, Sobol AM, Deronimus A. "Reducing Infant Mortality in Rural America: Evaluation of the Rural Infant Care Program." *Health Services Research* 1987; 22:104, 105. Copyright © 1987 by the Health Research and Educational Trust. Reprinted with permission of the Health Research and Educational Trust.

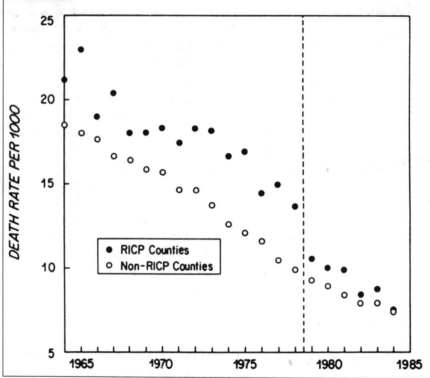

threats to internal validity. That is, if an external event occurred simultaneously with the program and caused an increase between O_4 and O_5, the event also likely would be experienced by the comparison group between O_{12} and O_{13}. If the increase between O_4 and O_5 was greater than the increase between O_{12} and O_{13}, the change could be attributed to the program, *provided that the comparison group is similar to the intervention group.* Thus, the addition of a comparison group introduces selection threats to internal validity, which may or may not be controlled, depending on the similarity of the two groups.

Multiple time series designs appear frequently in publications evaluating the impacts of health programs. For example, Gortmaker and associates (1987) used the design to determine the impact of a program to improve perinatal care

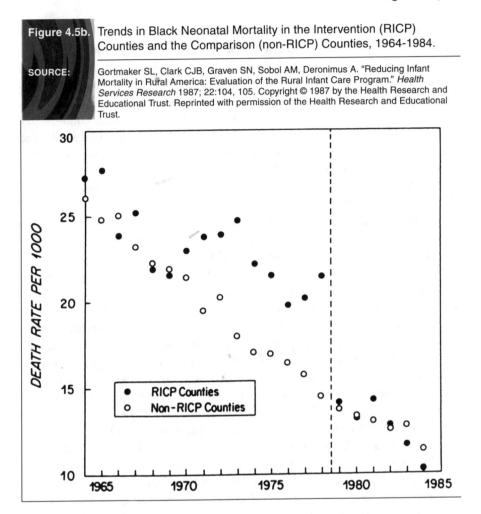

Figure 4.5b. Trends in Black Neonatal Mortality in the Intervention (RICP) Counties and the Comparison (non-RICP) Counties, 1964-1984.

SOURCE: Gortmaker SL, Clark CJB, Graven SN, Sobol AM, Deronimus A. "Reducing Infant Mortality in Rural America: Evaluation of the Rural Infant Care Program." *Health Services Research* 1987; 22:104, 105. Copyright © 1987 by the Health Research and Educational Trust. Reprinted with permission of the Health Research and Educational Trust.

on neonatal mortality rates in 10 rural counties with histories of high infant mortality. The comparison group consisted of urban and rural counties with "average" infant mortality rates, which represented a "performance standard" for gauging the success of the program. That is, if the high infant mortality rates in the program counties declined to levels similar to those in the average comparison counties, the program would be deemed a "success." Figure 4.5a compares neonatal mortality rates in the 10 program counties with neonatal rates in the comparison counties for 1964-1984. A sharp drop in neonatal mortality is observed in 1979, the year when the program counties began to plan and implement the intervention. A similar, even sharper decline in black neonatal mortality rates is observed in Figure 4.5b.

Similarly, Wagenaar (1981, 1986) used a multiple time series design to determine whether Michigan's increase in the legal drinking age from 18 to 21 in 1978 lowered traffic accidents. Using a 20% random sample of reported motor vehicle crashes, the treatment group was a monthly time series of alcohol-related crashes for drivers aged 18-20. Three comparison groups were constructed: (a) separate measures of alcohol-related and nonalcohol-related crashes for drivers aged 18-20, (b) all crashes for drivers aged 21-24, and (c) all crashes for drivers aged 25-45. Findings revealed that the law reduced alcohol-related crashes for drivers aged 18-20 by about 18% in the 12 months following the passage of the law, and a similar 16% reduction was detected 6 years after the law was passed.

Loftin and associates (1991) used the design to evaluate whether the District of Columbia's 1976 law banning the purchase, sale, transfer, or possession of handguns reduced firearm-related homicides and suicides. The comparison group was adjacent metropolitan areas in Maryland and Virginia. Four outcome measures captured the role of firearms in homicides and suicides: homicides per month by firearms, homicides per month by other means, suicides per month by firearms, and suicides per month by other means. By separating firearm-related deaths from nonfirearm-related deaths, the evaluators were in a stronger position to make causal inferences about the impacts of the law. Results indicated an abrupt decline in homicides and suicides by firearms after the law was implemented. No reductions were observed for homicides and suicides committed by other means, nor were there similar reductions in the comparison areas, and nor were there increases in homicides and suicides by other means.

Pierce and associates (1998) also used the design to determine whether the California Tobacco Control Program had reduced smoking in the state. The California Tobacco Control Program began in 1989, and the time series evaluation compared annual per capita cigarette consumption in California, with per capita rates in the United States as the comparison group. Although per capita consumption declined in both groups after 1989, the decline was greater in California than in the United States, particularly in the initial 3 years after the program started.

By adding a comparison group, all these studies improved the certainty of causal inferences that observed changes were due to the program rather than to other factors.

Repeated Treatment Design

In some cases, a program may have an effect, but if the program is removed or discontinued, the effect will disappear. If a program's effects are transitory, the repeated treatment design can be utilized to evaluate its impacts. Similar to a single time series, the repeated treatment design introduces and removes the intervention repeatedly. The design is diagramed below, where X indicates the intervention is introduced and –X indicates the intervention is removed (Cook and Campbell 1979; Reichardt and Mark 1998):

$$O_1 \; O_2 \; O_3 \; X \; O_4 \; O_5 \; O_6 \; -X \; O_7 \; O_8 \; O_9 \; X \; O_{10} \; O_{11} \; O_{12} \; -X \; O_{13} \; O_{14} \; O_{15}$$

Confidence in causal inferences about program effects is greater if O_3 differs from O_4, O_9 differs from O_{10}, and the $O_3 - O_4$ difference has the same direction and magnitude as the $O_9 - O_{10}$ difference. The design controls for history threats because external events are unlikely to have the same pattern of decreases and increases associated with the introduction and removal of the program. Like the single time series, instrumentation remains a possible threat, as well as attrition. The design should be used only for programs not affected by cyclical or seasonal factors. The design may be subject to Hawthorne effects if people in the intervention group become sensitive to the repeated introduction and removal of the intervention. In particular, if the intervention is desirable, people in the intervention group may become demoralized when it is withdrawn, and therefore changes may be due to the feelings and attitudes of participants rather than to the program itself.

The repeated treatment design rarely is used to evaluate the impacts of health programs, perhaps because of reluctance to withdraw an intervention with known health benefits. Schnelle and colleagues (1978) used the design to determine whether police helicopter surveillance, as an adjunct to patrol car surveillance, would decrease home burglaries in high crime areas. They found that when the helicopter surveillance was introduced, burglary rates fell, as shown in Figure 4.6. When helicopter surveillance was removed, burglary rates increased. The investigators repeated the introduction and removal of helicopter surveillance, and the same pattern of effects was observed.

Pretest-Posttest Nonequivalent Comparison Group Design

Suppose that you want to evaluate the impacts of the health promotion class to older adults in a clinic using the pretest-posttest control group design described earlier. The clinic director and staff, however, want to offer the program to all older adults in the clinic, and therefore randomization is not possible. As an alternative, you decide to evaluate the program using the *pretest-posttest nonequivalent comparison group design*, which is diagramed as follows (Camp-

Figure 4.6. Repeated Treatment Design: Daily Frequency of Home Burglaries With and Without Police Helicopter Surveillance[a]

SOURCE: Schnelle JF, Kirchner RE, Macrae JW, McNess MP, Eck RH, Snodgrass S, Casey JD, Uselton PH Jr. "Police Evaluation Research: An Experimental and Cost-Benefit Analysis of a Helicopter Patrol in a High-Crime Area." *Journal of Applied Behavior Analysis* 1978; 11:15.

a. Arrows indicate days helicopter was prevented from flying.

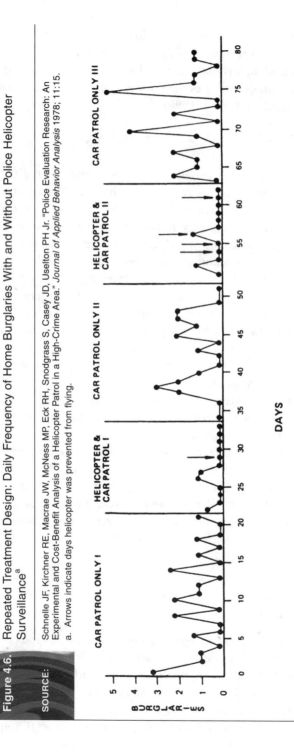

bell and Stanley 1963; Cook and Campbell 1979; Mohr 1995; Reichardt and Mark 1998; Rog 1994; Shortell and Richardson 1978):

$$O_1 \ X \ O_2$$
$$------$$
$$O_3 \quad O_4$$

The top row indicates the observations for the intervention group. The absence of Rs and the dashed line indicate that older adults were not randomized, and, therefore, the O_3 and O_4 observations are for a comparison group and not a true control group. A comparison group for the health promotion class might be older adults at another clinic with similar characteristics.

Because cases are not randomized to the intervention and control groups, selection is the main threat to internal validity in this design. Selection threats can be reduced but not eliminated by choosing a comparison group that is similar to the intervention group, matching cases in the intervention group with similar cases from the comparison population, and controlling statistically for baseline differences in the two groups through analysis of covariance (described in more detail in Chapter 9). For example, suppose the comparison group is formed by matching the demographic characteristics of people in the intervention group with those in the comparison group, and that after matching no statistically significant differences exist between groups for those demographic characteristics. Does this mean selection is no longer problem? Although the lack of statistically significant differences increases our confidence that the two groups are similar, the groups may still be different, for example, if the intervention group is composed of people who volunteered for the program. In this case, motivational differences exist between the two groups that are not controlled by matching, and internal validity may be threatened by the interaction of selection-history, selection-maturation, or selection-testing. For example, volunteers may have more motivation and enthusiasm, resulting in exposure to different historical events, a faster pace of learning, and greater sensitivity to pretest observations than people in the comparison group. When present, these selection interactions, rather than the program itself, may account for observed differences between groups.

Selection threats also can be reduced by using gain score analysis to control for baseline differences between the two groups (Reichardt and Mark 1998). For example, suppose that the O_1 average health knowledge score for the intervention group is 15 points higher than the O_3 average knowledge score for the comparison group, and that the intervention group would remain 15 points ahead at the posttest, except for the effect of the program. By computing the difference between the posttest and pretest scores for the two groups, gain scores adjust for the baseline selection differences between the groups. Gain score analysis does not, however, control for selection interactions, such as the interaction of selection and maturation, where one group improves faster than the other group even in the absence of the program.

Regression threats to internal validity also may apply to this design. If people in the intervention group are matched with people in the comparison group based on demographic characteristics, there may be individuals in either group with extremely low or high scores on the pretest, which will naturally regress toward the population mean on the posttest. In this case, the change between the pretest and posttest observations is due to regression toward the population mean and not the program itself.

In summary, the greater the similarity between the intervention and comparison groups, the greater confidence that observed differences between groups are due to the program and not to other factors. Regression and the self-selection of individuals into the intervention group become less important threats to internal validity if the intervention and comparison groups are two more or less natural groups, both of which are seeking and are eligible for the program. The group first receiving the program becomes the intervention group, and the other group, matched on demographic characteristics, becomes the comparison group. Because both groups have similar motivations, selection interaction and regression threats are reduced. Once the program is under way, however, the design remains subject to compensatory equalization of treatments, compensatory rivalry, resentful demoralization, and diffusion or imitation of treatments.

The pretest-posttest nonequivalent comparison group design is used often to evaluate the impacts of health programs. For example, Cherkin and colleagues (1989) used the design to evaluate the impact of a $5 copayment on office visits in Group Health Cooperative of Puget Sound. The intervention group, which faced a $5 copayment for each office visit, was composed of state government enrollees at Group Health. The comparison group, which did not face the copayment, consisted of a similar group of public employees, federal government enrollees at Group Health. As expected, the copayment decreased primary care and specialty care visits by different amounts.

Recurrent Institutional Cycle ("Patched-Up") Design

Suppose the health promotion class for older adults can accommodate a maximum of 20 people per class, and that more than 200 adults at the clinic want to take the class. You decide to offer the class several times over the coming year so that everyone can attend. When programs are repeated in "cycles" such as this, their impacts can be evaluated using the recurrent institutional cy-cle design, which is diagrammed as follows (Campbell and Stanley 1963; Cook and Campbell 1979; Shortell and Richardson 1978):

$$\begin{array}{c} X\ O_1 \\ \overline{} \\ O_2\ X\ O_3 \\ \overline{} \\ O_4 \end{array}$$

Each row in the design represents a cycle of the program, in this case a class of older adults. The top row indicates the O_1 posttest observation for adults just completing the class, the middle row indicates the O_2 pretest and posttest ob-servations for the next class, and the bottom row represents the pretest obser-vation (O_4) for the third class. The O_1 and the O_2 observations are made at ap-proximately the same time, and the O_3 and the O_4 observations also are made at about the same time. The lack of Rs and the dashed lines indicate that cases are not randomized to cycles. If big values mean good outcomes and statistical tests show that $O_1 > O_2$, $O_3 > O_2$, and $O_3 > O_4$, observed outcomes are likely due to the program and not to other factors. Because causal inferences depend on a complex pattern of outcomes, Cook and Campbell (1979) recommend that large samples and reliable measures be used to reduce the likelihood that outcomes are due to chance.

If one or more of these patterns are not found, observed outcomes may be due to other factors, which may be understood by reviewing the design's threats to internal validity. The institutional cycle design is really an assembly of the three pre-experimental designs described earlier in this chapter. The top row ($X\ O_1$) is the *one-group posttest-only design*, and its major threats to inter-nal validity are history and maturation. The middle row ($O_2\ X\ O_3$) is the *sin-gle group pretest-posttest design*, which is vulnerable to history, matura-tion, testing, instrumentation, and regression threats. The top and middle rows ($\begin{array}{c} X\ O_1 \\ \overline{} \\ O_2 \end{array}$) form the *posttest-only comparison group design*, which is subject to attrition and selection threats. Similarly, the middle and bottom rows ($\begin{array}{c} X\ O_3 \\ \overline{} \\ O_4 \end{array}$)

also form the posttest-only comparison group design. Although each design has multiple threats to internal validity, when they are "patched" together, a num-ber of threats may be controlled. As shown in Table 4.3, the posttest-only com-parison group design controls for history threats, which are not controlled by the one-group posttest-only design and the pretest-posttest design. In addition, the posttest-only comparison group design controls for threats from testing and instrumentation in the pretest-posttest design. In the same way, the pretest-posttest design controls for selection threats, which are a problem with the posttest-only comparison group design.

The design does not, however, control for maturation, regression, and attrition. Maturation threats are a less serious problem in relatively short health education programs, where there is less opportunity for subjects to change internally in ways that also might account for program outcomes. In contrast, if the program's aim is to increase health status, maturation threats may exist, as described earlier in the single group pretest-posttest design. Regression threats may exist if exposure to the program is prioritized based on extreme scores. For example, if the sickest people received the program first, they would have better health at the posttest simply due to regression to the mean. Attrition threats also apply, for the number and characteristics of people who drop out can be different in each cycle of the program.

As described earlier, the institutional cycle design may be applied when the program is offered on a regular cycle, and when the administration of a pretest to the group of individuals waiting for the next cycle is not feasible (if a pretest is feasible, the pretest-posttest nonequivalent comparison group design also may be used). The institutional cycle design also has been used to evaluate the performance of the health care system. For example, Diehr and her associates (1979) examined the impact of prepaid health care on health status among low-income families. The first intervention group consisted of 748 people enrolled into the program in 1973. The second cycle of the program consisted of 941 individuals enrolled into the program in 1974. In addition, another, different group of 1,649 people enrolled in 1971 were followed for selected measures. This "patched-up" design works well because of its close "fit" with the natural implementation of the program and because many threats to internal validity are controlled.

In summary, the institutional cycle design is well suited for ongoing programs where people or other cases cycle through them in a repetitive manner. Because some threats are not controlled with the design, and because causal inferences of program effects hinge on finding a complex pattern of outcomes, the design is not a strong one but may be the only one suitable for a specific context.

Regression Discontinuity Design

Returning to the previous example, suppose you are launching a health promotion program for older adults who had more than 10 physician visits in the previous year. Older adults with 10 or more physician visits receive the program, and older adults with 9 or fewer visits do not receive the program. One year later, information about the health knowledge of older adults in the two groups is collected through telephone interviews. If a program has a "cut-point" or "threshold," where people at or above the cut-point receive the program and those below it do not, the program's effects can be estimated through the regression discontinuity design (Campbell and Stanley 1963; Cook and Campbell 1979; Marcantonio and Cook 1994; Reichardt and Mark 1998; Shortell and Richardson 1978; Trochim 1990).

Figure 4.7 illustrates the design, which is more a type of statistical analysis than an experimental design. The graph's x-axis is the quantitative score—in this case, annual physician visits, indicating eligibility for the program. A vertical line indicates the cut-point of 10 visits in the prior year, which is known as the "quantitative assignment variable," or QAV (Reichardt and Mark 1998). The y-axis is the program's outcome, which in this case is a health knowledge score, calculated for each person from the information collected in the telephone interview. Each person's number of physician visits is plotted against that person's health knowledge score. The resulting regression line indicates the relationship between physician visits and health knowledge scores. If a statistically significant break, or "discontinuity," is detected *at the cut-point*, we can infer that the program increased health knowledge in persons above the cut-point.

The regression discontinuity design controls for most threats to internal validity. History and maturation are controlled because both groups were considered for the program at the same time and were followed for the same length of time. Testing is usually not a threat because both groups are exposed to the same procedure for determining eligibility for the program. Instrumentation is usually controlled because the instrument for measuring outcomes is applied to both groups. Instrumentation threats might occur, however, if the agency conducting the program also did the follow-up assessments. In this case, gratitude for receiving the program and resentment for being denied entry into the program may affect self-reports of health knowledge in either a positive or a negative direction. This potential problem can be eliminated by having another agency perform the follow-ups. Regression and selection may exist but can be ruled out as alternative explanations of program effects. That is, selection and regression are evident because only persons above a cut-point were selected into the program. If, however, a break is detected at the cut-point, where the two groups are similar, the difference is not explained by the selection factors themselves. Attrition is a potential problem if the follow-up response rates are higher in the group receiving the program than the group that does not. This may occur, for example, if the agency running the program also does the follow-up in-

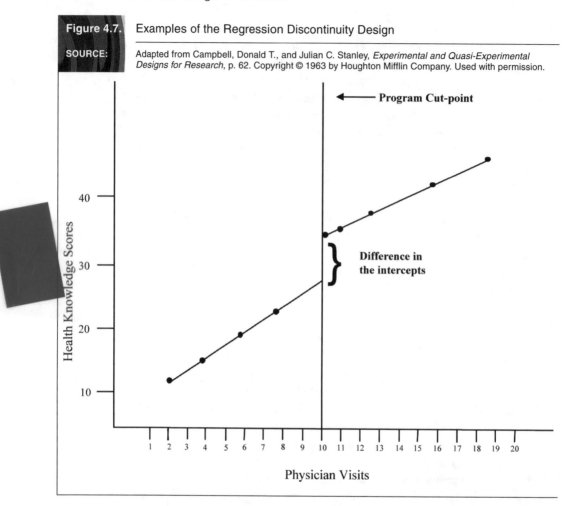

Figure 4.7. Examples of the Regression Discontinuity Design

SOURCE: Adapted from Campbell, Donald T., and Julian C. Stanley, *Experimental and Quasi-Experimental Designs for Research*, p. 62. Copyright © 1963 by Houghton Mifflin Company. Used with permission.

terviews. This problem can be reduced by having an independent agency conduct the interviews. Selection-interaction threats are controlled if they cannot explain the discontinuity in the regression line at the cut-point.

Finally, if the program is highly desirable, withholding the program from people below the cut-point may result in resentful demoralization, which might affect follow-up responses in ways that explain the discontinuity in the regression line at the cut-point. For example, if persons denied entry into the program are resentful or demoralized, their feelings may alter their responses in the follow-up interview toward revealing less health knowledge than they actually possess, which may account for the discontinuity at the cut-point, rather than the program itself accounting for it.

The design controls for some threats to external validity. Testing-treatment interaction is controlled to the extent that eligibility for the program is always defined by a cut-point. Selection-treatment interaction does pose a threat because the effect has been demonstrated only for those clustered at the cut-point, and effects may not apply to other groups. Setting and history interaction effects may pose a problem, for example, if program effects are observed in a clinic but disappear when the program is implemented in other settings. Multiple treatment effects may be a threat if those above the cut-point also are participating in other programs.

The regression discontinuity design also can be applied to determine the effectiveness of new medical treatments, where patients must surpass a severity-of-illness threshold to receive the new treatment, as shown in Figure 4.8 (Marcantonio and Cook 1994). Using hypothetical data, the x-axis presents the initial severity of illness for 200 patients, where low scores indicate greater severity. Those below the cut-point of 50 receive the new medical treatment, while those above the cut-point receive standard care. The y-axis indicates posttreatment severity of illness. The discontinuity in the regression line at the cut-point indicates a treatment affect. The new treatment (experimental) group members have higher posttreatment scores, which indicate less severity of illness, than the group receiving usual care.

In summary, the regression discontinuity design is a strong one but is applied infrequently to evaluate the impact of health programs. Perhaps the best known examples are Lohr (1972) and Wilder (1972), who employed the design to determine the impact of the Medicaid program on physician visits, where families below a low income threshold were eligible for the program, and those above the threshold were not. In addition, Mellor and Mark (1998) have applied the design to evaluate the impacts of administrative decisions based on cutoff scores.

This concludes the review of pre-experimental, quasi-experimental, and experimental designs on the internal validity continuum in Figure 4.2. None of the designs controls for all threats to internal validity, and external validity is highly questionable across all designs as well. Furthermore, political issues from Act I of the evaluation process may influence the choice of impact design in Act II. For example, Morris (1998) describes a political "hot potato" where the agency director asks the evaluator to replace the evaluation's randomized impact design with another design to appease interest groups, who believe it is "patently unfair" to deprive people of a service that would benefit them. There are no simple solutions to this ethical, political, and methodological dilemma. Eastmond (1998) and Scheirer (1998) illustrate how an alternative design could

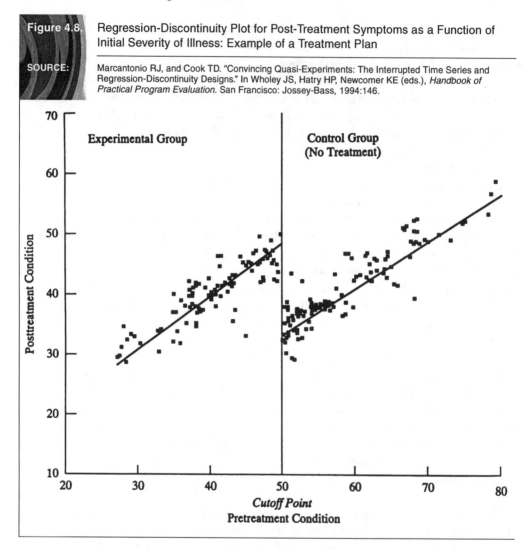

Figure 4.8.   Regression-Discontinuity Plot for Post-Treatment Symptoms as a Function of Initial Severity of Illness: Example of a Treatment Plan

SOURCE: Marcantonio RJ, and Cook TD. "Convincing Quasi-Experiments: The Interrupted Time Series and Regression-Discontinuity Designs." In Wholey JS, Hatry HP, Newcomer KE (eds.), *Handbook of Practical Program Evaluation*. San Francisco: Jossey-Bass, 1994:146.

be chosen by applying the Guiding Principles for Evaluators (American Evaluation Association 1995).

STATISTICAL AND MEASUREMENT THREATS

To infer that outcomes are due to the program and not to other factors, a statistically significant association must exist between the program and the outcome. This section presents threats to "statistical conclusion validity," or characteristics of the program evaluation that may reduce the likelihood of detecting a statistically significant program effect, if such an effect in fact exists (Cook and Campbell 1979). A related concern, measurement reliability, also is described.

Low Statistical Power

If the number of cases in the intervention or control group is too small, the statistical test may indicate that the program has no effect when in fact one actually exists. In short, if sample sizes are small or alpha (α) is low, there is an increased risk of making a Type II error, or inferring that the program has no impact when in fact one actually exists. Methods for calculating minimum sample sizes that eliminate this problem are presented in Chapter 7.

Violated Assumptions of Statistical Tests

Statistical tests for estimating program effects have assumptions that must be met to make accurate interpretations of test results. For example, a program may be designed to increase access to health services, and expenditures for health services is one outcome measure of the program. In most populations, health expenditures do not have a normal distribution (Duan et al. 1983), which is often required by many statistical tests. In most cases this problem can be overcome by either transforming the observations to create a normal distribution or choosing an alternative statistical procedure that has different assumptions about the distribution of the data.

Fishing and Error Rate Problem

Many health programs have several outcome measures. For example, a health promotion program may be implemented to increase the health knowledge of participants. The outcome measure is a self-administered instrument containing 20 true/false questions about health care. When each item is compared for people in the program versus the control group, a statistically significant difference will be obtained for one of the items by chance alone. This is known as a Type I error, or concluding that the program has an effect when in fact one does not exist. The "fishing and error rate" problem occurs when the intervention and control groups are compared across several measures, a small number of comparisons are statistically significant by chance alone, and the evaluator incorrectly concludes that the program has beneficial effects.

Reliability of Program Implementation

If a program is implemented in different schools, clinics, communities, or other settings, implementation may differ across sites. In addition, when a program is delivered to people, the delivery may differ across people. As the variation in program implementation increases, error variance also increases, which decreases the likelihood of detecting a program effect. The solution to this problem is to standardize the delivery of the program as much as possible across persons and sites.

Random Irrelevancies in the Program Setting

When a program is implemented, an unplanned event may occur in the environment that may affect observed outcomes. For example, suppose you are evaluating the effect of managed care on health expenditures in a state. During the course of data collection, the state legislature imposes new regulations on managed care firms, which may affect future expenditures. Environmental changes, such as new state regulations, inflate variation and decrease the likelihood of detecting a program effect. Although this problem cannot be eliminated, it can be addressed, when feasible, by measuring the magnitude of the changes and controlling for them in the statistical analysis.

Random Heterogeneity of Respondents

Suppose you wanted to reduce head injuries from bicycle accidents among children. You secure funds to offer bicycle helmets at half price to preschool and elementary school children in the city. Even at half price, however, some low-income families who want to buy helmets for their children may not have resources to do so. In this case, one of the program's outcomes, the number of children with helmets in the city, will vary, depending on family income. When people exposed to the program have different characteristics that are correlated with the outcome measure, error variance is inflated, which reduces the likelihood of observing a program effect. This problem can be controlled, in this case, by stratified sampling based on income, or including income as a covariate in the statistical analysis.

Measurement Reliability

Another potential threat to internal validity is the reliability of outcome measures, or measurement error (Green and Lewis 1986). A program may have a valid underlying theory of cause and effect, and it may be implemented well in the field (see Chapter 3). The statistical analysis, however, may reveal no program effects. The failure to detect a program effect when one actually exists, or Type II error problem, may occur when the measures of program outcomes are unreliable. The problem occurs because unreliability inflates standard errors of estimates, which reduce the likelihood of detecting a program effect, if one in fact exists. This problem can be reduced by employing outcome measures with known reliability, validity, and sensitivity in detecting differences between groups, which will be discussed in more detail in Chapter 8.

EVALUATION OF IMPACT DESIGNS AND META-ANALYSIS

The preceding review of impact designs reveals an important fact: Uncertainty is an inherent feature of impact evaluation. All designs for evaluating the impacts of health programs are subject to one or more threats to internal validity; therefore, in any given impact evaluation, uncertainty exists about whether observed outcomes are due to the program or to other factors. Two types of errors in making causal inference are possible: (a) inferring that the program has an effect when it actually does not (Type I error) and (b) inferring that the program has no effect when it actually does (Type II error). More than one design can be applied to estimate the impacts of most health programs, and the goal is to choose the design that reduces the likelihood of making either error when drawing causal inferences of program effects.

Thus, the choice of impact design is a key decision in the evaluation process. In principle, because randomized designs have the fewest threats to internal validity and therefore the lowest likelihood of Type I and II errors, they are preferred in programs where randomization is feasible. Although internal validity threats can be reduced in nonrandomized designs, for example by matching cases in the intervention and comparison groups based on characteristics that can be measured (such as age and gender), the two groups may still have different unmeasured characteristics (such as motivation and attitudes) that may account for observed outcomes.

To test this proposition, "evaluations of impact evaluations" have been conducted to determine whether different impact designs yield similar or different estimates of program effects. Campbell and Boruch (1975) examined evaluations of educational programs and found that nonrandomized designs underestimated program effects, relative to randomized designs. Deniston and Rosenstock (1973) estimated the effects of an arthritis control program using three alternative designs. Relative to the randomized design, the pretest-posttest design overestimated program effects, while the nonequivalent comparison group design underestimated program effects. Friedlander and Robins (1994) estimated the effects of four randomized welfare-to-work programs in Baltimore, Arkansas, Virginia, and San Diego. Using data from the four sites, they estimated program effects using a variety of nonequivalent comparison groups. For example, the intervention group in one site was compared with the three control groups from the three other sites. They also estimated program effects with and without controlling statistically for differences in personal characteristics between groups. Program effects varied greatly and had opposite signs across the different comparison groups (Rossi 1997). In contrast to these findings, Aiken and associates (1998) compared the program effects of a remedial writing program for university freshmen using three designs (randomized experiment, nonequivalent control group, and regression discontinuity) and found similar effects. As a whole, these findings suggest that different estimates of program effects usually are obtained with randomized and nonequivalent comparison group designs.

The influence of the evaluation methods on estimates of program effects also has been examined using meta-analysis, a quantitative technique for synthesizing program effects across several studies (Cordray and Fischer 1994). Lipsey (1997), Wilson (1995), and Lipsey and Wilson (1993) examined the mean effect sizes of more than 300 psychological, behavioral, and educational interventions. They found that a large percentage of the individual studies found no positive effects due to small sample sizes. The interventions, however, generally had positive effects when the sample sizes of all the studies were combined in the meta-analysis. They also found that about 25% of the variation in effect sizes across studies was due to the program itself, about 21% was due to study methods (sample size and the types of design, control group, and measures), about 26% was due to sampling error, and the remaining 28% was residual or unexplained variation. Lipsey (1992) conducted a similar meta-analysis of delinquency intervention studies, and the four sources accounted for similar percentages of the variation in effect size across studies. These findings also indicate that different impact designs yield different estimates of program effects. They also indicate that low sample size is an important threat to statistical conclusion validity.

The review of impact designs also reveals a second, important fact: External validity threats exist in all impact designs, and therefore, findings from a single impact evaluation usually cannot be generalized to other populations and settings. The generalizability of program effects can be improved by including diverse target groups from a variety of settings in the intervention and control groups. When this is not possible, generalizability can be assessed by replicating the program in diverse settings and populations. After several individual evaluations of the program are completed, meta-analysis can be conducted to examine the variation in program effects across the studies and to estimate the average size of program effects (Cook 1993). The latter strategy was followed in the Medicare COBRA demonstrations described in Chapter 3, where the cost-effectiveness of preventive services for Medicare enrollees was evaluated in six sites. The data from the sites were combined into a single data set to examine intervention effects across sites and to estimate the average effect sizes.

SUMMARY

In Act I of the evaluation process, decision makers and interest groups typically ask questions about the impacts of health programs. A key decision in Act II of the evaluation process is the choice of an impact design to answer those questions. Alternative impact designs exist, each having its own strengths and weaknesses. The goal is to choose a design that is feasible and fits well with logistical, political, budget, and other constraints of the program, and that has the fewest threats to internal validity that can undermine causal inferences about program effects. If an impact design is chosen that has one or more threats to internal validity, evaluators often can improve their understanding of the magnitude and importance of the threats by collecting information about the implementation of the program, as described in Chapter 6.

Once an impact design is chosen, decision makers may want to know about the benefits of a program as well as the costs of producing them. Methods for answering questions about the costs and effects of health programs are reviewed in the next chapter.

LIST OF TERMS _____

Causal inference
Design threats to internal validity
   Attrition
   Field threats
      Ambiguity about the direction of causal inference
      Compensatory equalization of treatments
      Compensatory rivalry by people receiving less desirable treatments
      Diffusion or imitation of program
      Resentful demoralization of respondents receiving less
         desirable treatments
   History
   Instrumentation
   Interaction threats
      Selection-history
      Selection-maturation
   Maturation
   Regression
   Selection
   Testing
  External validity
  Impact designs
   Experimental
      Posttest-only control group
      Pretest-posttest control group
      Solomon four-group
   Pre-experimental
      One group pretest-posttest
      One-shot case study
      Posttest-only comparison group
   Quasi-experimental
      Institutional cycle
      Multiple time series
      Nonequivalent control group
      Regression discontinuity
      Repeated treatments
      Single time series
  Internal validity
  Measurement reliability

Meta-analysis
Statistical conclusion threats to internal validity
    Fishing and error rate problem
    Low statistical power
    Random heterogeneity of respondents
    Random irrelevancies in program setting
    Reliability of program implementation
    Violated assumptions
Threats to external validity
    Interaction threats
        History-treatment
        Selection-treatment
        Setting-treatment (reactive effects)
        Testing-treatment
    Multiple treatments

STUDY QUESTIONS

1. What are the requirements for making causal inferences in an impact evaluation?

2. What is the difference between the definitions of internal and external validity?

3. What are the seven major threats to internal validity?

4. What is meant by "statistical conclusion validity"?

5. Why is it important to use valid and reliable measures in impact evaluation?

6. What are the names of the different impact designs described in this chapter? If you had to describe each design to a friend, how would you do so?

7. What factors should an evaluator consider in choosing an impact design for a program?

8. Are experimental designs always better than quasi-experimental designs?

9. What can an evaluator do if an impact design fails (that is, the design is not implemented as intended in the field)?

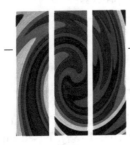

CHAPTER 5

Cost-Effectiveness Analysis

To judge the worth of a program, funding agencies, program administrators, and other interest groups decide to conduct an impact evaluation of a program in Act I of the evaluation process. In the course of doing so, they realize that all programs entail costs but may or may not produce expected benefits. If the program does not have good outcomes, they might decide that the program is not worth the costs of implementing it. On the other hand, if the program works, they may want to know how much it costs to obtain its benefits. This question is particularly important to the funding agency because it has limited resources to devote to the program. In the agency's view, a program that produces more benefits with a limited budget is worth more than an alternative program that produces fewer benefits with the same budget, other things equal. In short, the worth of a program is judged more stringently: The program must have beneficial outcomes *and* produce them at least cost.

In practice, the decision to conduct an impact evaluation is actually made in response to a two-part question: Does the program actually produce expected benefits, and if so, at what cost? Cost-effectiveness analysis is the most common approach in health program evaluation for answering the second question. Although the concept of cost-effectiveness analysis is relatively simple, the application of the concepts is often complicated (Warner 1989). In the next section, the concept of cost-effectiveness analysis is defined. Next, methods are presented for comparing the costs and effects of programs through cost-effectiveness ratios. The third section reviews the basic types of cost-effectiveness analysis, and the fourth section presents the basic steps of designing and conducting a cost-effectiveness analysis. The final section summarizes some key points about conducting a cost-effectiveness analysis in the evaluation process.

COST-EFFECTIVENESS ANALYSIS: AN AID TO DECISION MAKING

A major reason for performing a cost-effectiveness analysis (CEA) is to rationalize the allocation of scarce health care resources (Warner 1989). Based on the principles of welfare economics, the basic premises of CEA are that (Fuchs 1974; Garber et al. 1996)

1. health care resources are scarce,
2. resources have alternative uses,
3. people have different wants, and
4. there are never enough resources to satisfy all wants.

The key economic challenge, therefore, is deciding how to allocate scarce resources efficiently to satisfy human wants. The purpose of CEA is to help decision makers judge the *relative efficiency* of alternative ways of achieving a desired benefit to guide their allocations of resources (Urban 1998). A strategy is "efficient" if no other strategy is as effective at lower cost. When used properly, CEA is a useful tool that can help decision makers compare the cost and outcome trade-offs between alternative ways of allocating scarce resources. Given desired outcomes, CEA can identify the least-cost alternative for achieving those outcomes or, conversely, how to achieve the most outcomes with a fixed budget (Warner 1989).

CEA, however, is *not* a decision-*making* technique. The findings from a CEA do not determine which alternative to choose over others. Those trade-offs inevitably entail value judgments about the worth of program outcomes and the cost of producing them, which only decision makers can make (Petitti 1994; Warner 1989). To illustrate this important point, Warner and Luce (1982) and Warner (1989) describe two hypothetical programs. Program A costs $100,000 and saves 12 lives; the average cost per life saved is $8,333. Program B costs $200,000 and saves 15 lives; its average cost per life saved is $13,333. Because Program A's average costs are lower than those of Program B, Program A might appear to be the "better" program. By spending an additional $100,000, however, Program B saves 3 more lives than does Program A. The incremental cost for each additional life saved is $33,333 ($100,000/3). This leads to the fundamental question: Is saving an additional 3 lives worth the additional $100,000? CEA cannot answer this question because it entails judgments of worth based on human values.

CEA is one of four types of economic evaluation to compare the costs and outcomes of health programs. The names and descriptions of the other types of economic evaluation are presented below (Drummond et al. 1997). All three types of economic evaluation are capable of evaluating the costs and outcomes of two or more programs.

> *Cost-benefit analysis (CBA):* A method of economic evaluation where all benefits and costs of a program are measured in dollars. Programs have value when their benefits are equal to or exceed their costs, or the ratio of $benefits/$costs is equal to or greater than 1.0, or when the benefit/cost ratio of Program A is equal to or greater than 1.0 and exceeds the benefit/cost ratio of Program B.
>
> *Cost-minimization analysis (CMA):* A type of cost-effectiveness analysis where Program A and Program B have identical outcomes, and the goal of the analysis is to determine which program has the lower costs.
>
> *Cost-utility analysis (CUA):* A type of cost-effectiveness analysis in which the outcomes of Program A and Program B are weighted by their value, or quality, and measured with a common metric, such as "quality-adjusted life years," and the goal of the analysis is to determine which program produces the most quality-adjusted life years at lower cost.

As the allocation of scarce resources has become more important in the U.S. health care system, so has the annual number of published cost-effectiveness (including cost-utility) studies in the literature, from 5 studies in 1966 to 518 studies in 1996 (Elixhauser et al. 1998). Between 1979 and 1996, 4,171 cost-benefit and cost-effectiveness studies were published. About 81% of the 2,274 studies published between 1991 and 1996 were cost-effectiveness/utility studies (Elixhauser et al. 1998), while the remainder were cost-benefit studies. Cost-effectiveness and cost-utility studies likely appear more frequently in the literature than do cost-benefit studies because the former studies do not require placing a dollar value on the intervention's benefits, such as years of life saved. One important question in cost-benefit analysis is how to value lives saved or lost due to a program, and different methods exist for performing this calculation. For example, in the evaluation of an HIV prevention program (Reid 2000), the value of a human life saved may be calculated by the future earnings approach (where the labor market determines the value of a person) or the required compensation approach (where people indicate how many dollars they require to risk the loss of their lives).

COMPARING PROGRAM COSTS AND EFFECTS: THE COST-EFFECTIVENESS RATIO

The basic goal of cost-effectiveness analysis is to compare the cost of a health program with its effectiveness (Warner 1989). One way of comparing costs and outcomes is simply to calculate the average cost of producing a benefit. For example, suppose that you are a maternity nurse in a hospital and teach prenatal care classes to pregnant women and their partners. Based on evidence in the literature and on observing the birth outcomes of women who attend your class, you realize that smoking is a risk factor for low birth weight, and you develop a program composed of counseling sessions and self-help materials to help pregnant smokers quit smoking (Floyd et al. 1993). Using a pretest-posttest design, you deliver the program to 100 pregnant smokers, and 25 women quit smoking. Based on hospital accounting records, the total costs of the program were $1,000; therefore, the average cost per quitter is $40 ($1,000/25 = $40).

Although calculating the average cost is informative, it does not help the nurse, hospital administrators, or other groups judge the worth of the program. With a pretest-posttest design, the impact evaluation observes only the quit rates among pregnant women who received the smoking cessation program. If the same 100 women had *not* received the smoking cessation program, some of the women likely would have quit smoking on their own. For example, let's assume that 10 out of 100 pregnant smokers would have quit smoking on their own without participating in the program and, therefore, the program has caused just an additional 15 pregnant smokers to quit smoking (25 – 10 = 15). The key cost-effectiveness question therefore may be stated as follows: *What are the additional costs of convincing 15 additional pregnant smokers to quit smoking, compared to pregnant smokers who do not receive the program?* If we assume that pregnant smokers who do not receive the smoking cessation program have zero program costs, the answer to this question is simply ($1,000 – $0)/(25 – 10) = $67 per quitter. In short, the core feature of a CEA is the *incremental* comparison of an intervention with an alternative (Garber et al. 1996; Torrance et al. 1996). This comparison, or *cost-effectiveness ratio (C/E*

Figure 5.1. Determining Whether a Program Is "Cost-Effective"

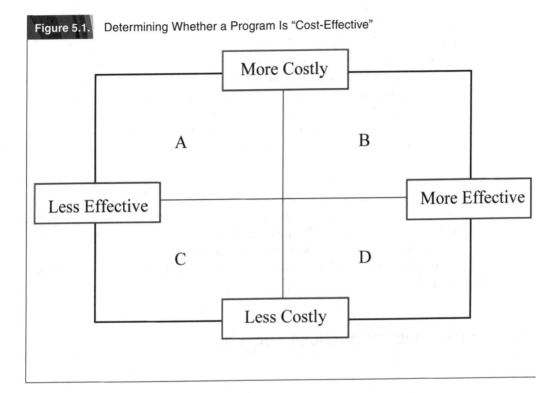

ratio), is a measure of the *incremental cost* of gaining an *incremental benefit* from a health program when compared with an alternative (Garber et al. 1996).

Whether a program is "cost-effective" depends on the relationship between program costs and effects, relative to an alternative, as shown in Figure 5.1 (Drummond et al. 1997; Petitti 1994). The vertical axis displays the relative costs of a program, compared to an alternative, ranging from more to less costly. The horizontal axis shows the relative effects of a program, ranging from less to more effective. A program that is less costly and at least as effective as the alternative falls into Quadrant D and is automatically "cost-effective" and should be adopted. In direct contrast, a program that is more costly and less effective falls into Quadrant A; this program is not cost-effective and should be rejected. A program in Quadrant B is more effective and more costly than the alternative, and the program is cost-effective *if* the added benefit is worth the added cost. A program in Quadrant C is less effective and less costly than the alternative, and the program is cost-effective *if* the added benefit of the alternative is not worth its added cost. CEA is recommended for programs in Quadrants B and C to help decision makers identify their relative merits, although health programs that fall into Quadrant C are rare (Doubilet et al. 1986; Drummond et al. 1997; Petitti 1994).

Programs also are cost-effective when they save costs and offer equal or better outcomes than the alternative (Doubilet et al. 1986; Petitti 1994; Warner 1989). Programs are cost-saving when they bring in more resources than they cost, which rarely happens in health care. When decision makers stipulate that a program must be cost-saving to have worth, they are imposing a more stringent requirement for judging the program's worth. As noted in Chapter 1, this is a particular problem for preventive programs when people believe that a dollar invested today to prevent disease should be offset by future savings in treatment costs. In fact, although few prevention programs are cost-saving (Russell 1993; Sisk 1993), many prevention programs are cost-effective when compared to therapeutic treatments (Phillips and Holtgrave 1997). For prevention programs, just like therapeutic programs, the real question may not be "How much does this program save?" but more simply "How much is this program worth?" (Huntington and Connell 1994).

TYPES OF COST-EFFECTIVENESS ANALYSIS

Cost-Effectiveness Studies of Health Programs

In general, cost-effectiveness evaluations can be divided into two broad types, which are similar to the types of health program evaluation defined in Chapter 1. The first type, *cost-effectiveness studies of health programs*, includes health programs created to reduce or eliminate a health problem or achieve a specific objective, such as water fluoridation to reduce caries, immunization programs to reduce the incidence of infectious diseases, or programs to increase healthy lifestyles.

Cost-effectiveness studies of health programs may be divided into the following three categories. The first category consists of studies in which a cost-effectiveness evaluation is conducted as part of an impact evaluation of a health program. For example, Windsor et al. (1985) used a randomized pretest-posttest control group design to determine the effectiveness of self-help smoking cessation interventions for pregnant smokers. As part of the randomized trial, Windsor et al. (1988) examined the cost-effectiveness of the self-help smoking cessation interventions. The results are presented in Table 5.1. Group 1 consisted of pregnant smokers who received the standard information in a "nonfocused," 5-minute interaction on smoking and pregnancy at the first prenatal visit.

TABLE 5.1 Cost-Effectiveness of Three Smoking Cessation Methods for Pregnant Smokers

Group	Cost per Patient	Percentage Who Quit	Average Cost-Effectiveness[d]	Incremental Cost-Effectiveness[e]
1. Standard information[a]	$2.08	2	$104.00	
2. American Lung Association manual[b]	$7.13	6	$118.83	$126.25
3. Pregnant Woman's Guide[c]	$7.13	14	$ 50.93	$ 42.08

SOURCE: Adapted from "A Cost-Effectiveness Analysis of Self-Help Smoking Cessation Methods for Pregnant Women," Windsor, Warner, and Cutter. © Copyright 1988 by Oxford University Press.

a. Group 1 was given information in a nonfocused interaction on smoking and pregnancy.
b. Group 2 received standard information plus the *Freedom From Smoking in 20 Days* manual of the American Lung Association.
c. Group 3 received standard information plus a self-help manual for pregnant women.
d. Cost-effectiveness = cost per patient/proportion who quit (effectiveness).
e. Relative to standard information.

Group 2 received the standard information *plus* a copy of *Freedom From Smoking in 20 Days*, published by the American Lung Association (ALA). Group 3 received the standard information *plus* a self-help manual designed specifically for pregnant smokers, *A Pregnant Woman's Self-Help Guide to Quit Smoking*.

The average cost-effectiveness of each intervention is simply the cost per patient divided by the percent who quit; for example, the average cost-effectiveness of the *Pregnant Woman's Guide* is $7.13/.14 = $50.93. The incremental cost-effectiveness of the ALA manual and the *Pregnant Woman's Guide* are calculated *relative* to the standard information benchmark. For example, when the formula for the incremental C/E ratio is applied, the $42.08 incremental cost-effectiveness of the *Pregnant Woman's Guide* is calculated as follows: ($7.13 – $2.08)/(.14 – .02) = $42.08. To interpret and understand the $42 incremental C/E ratio, let's assume that the standard information group consists of 100 pregnant smokers. The 2% quit rate indicates that 2 women quit smoking at $2.08 per woman, or $208 for the group. Let's also assume that the *Pregnant Woman's Guide* group consists of 100 pregnant smokers. The 14% quit rate indicates that 14 women quit at $7.13 per woman, or $713 for the group. The difference in the number of quitters between the two groups is 12 pregnant smokers (14 – 2 = 12), and the difference in the costs between the two group is $505 ($713 – $208 = $505). Dividing these two differences yields the incremental C/E ratio of about $42 ($505/12 = $42). In short, 12 more women quit smoking in the *Pregnant Woman's Guide* group than in the standard information group, and it costs $42 more for *each* additional woman to quit smoking.

The second category of cost-effectiveness evaluations of health programs consists of studies comparing the published results from two or more impact evaluations of a health program that appear in the literature. For example, Cummings et al. (1989) examined the cost-effectiveness of physician counseling to quit smoking during a routine office visit. Their cost-effectiveness analysis was based on the results from four published, randomized trials of brief advice to quit smoking, along with three randomized trials examining the impact of follow-up visits on quit rates. They found that the cost-effectiveness of brief advice during physician office visits ranged from $705 to $988 per year of life saved for men and from $1,204 to $2,058 for women (in 1984 dollars).

Similarly, Hatziandreu et al. (1995) examined the cost-effectiveness of three programs to increase use of bicycle helmets and reduce head injuries among children. In the first program, in Howard County, Maryland, a law was passed requiring bicyclists under age 16 to wear helmets. In the second program, in Seattle, Washington, a community-based approach was taken where public service announcements, community events, price discounts on bicycle helmets, and other measures were taken to increase helmet use. In the third program, in Oakland County, Mississippi, a school-based approach was taken to increase helmet use. A pretest-posttest design was used to estimate program effects in all three programs. Based on estimates of program costs and outcomes, the investigators concluded that the legislative and community measures had similar costs per injury avoided, but because the legislative program produced more immediate results than the community approach, the legislative program appeared to be the most cost-effective.

In short, if two or more impact evaluations of a health program appear in the published literature, a cost-effectiveness analysis may be feasible using secondary data from the studies, provided that the data required for calculating the C/E ratios are reported in the original studies. Compared to CEA that must await the completion of an impact evaluation, a CEA based on published impact evaluations can be conducted in less time, which is an advantage of this approach, *if* published impact evaluations of similar health programs exist in the literature.

The third category of cost-effectiveness studies of health programs consists of meta-analyses for quantitatively combining the results from several impact evaluations, mainly to improve the external validity, or generalizability, of the findings and thereby increase the relevance of the findings to decision making (Luce and Simpson 1995). For example, Hedrick et al. (1989) conducted a meta-analysis of the effects of home care on mortality among older adults. They examined 13 studies and found a small, beneficial effect of home care on mortality that fell short of statistical significance. In principle, if the effect of home care had been significant and positive, this finding could have been combined with estimates of home care costs to derive a C/E ratio of the cost per year of life gained due to home care. CEAs of health programs based on meta-analysis are relatively rare in the literature, mainly because typically there are not enough impact studies for many specific health programs and, therefore, results cannot be combined in the meta-analysis (Hedrick et al. 1989).

Cost-Effectiveness Evaluations of Health Services

The second broad category of cost-effectiveness evaluation consists of *cost-effectiveness studies comparing the costs and outcomes of one health service with another* (Garber et al. 1996). Fuchs (1986) describes the essence of the economic question. As shown in Figure 5.2, when a patient receives a health service, health status tends to rise sharply with initial treatment, where small additional amounts of care are associated with great increases in health (point C). At some point, however, the rate of increase in health begins to level

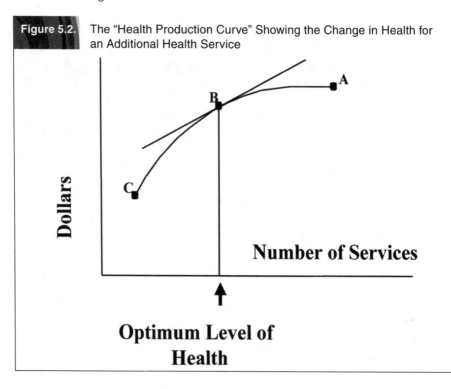

Figure 5.2. The "Health Production Curve" Showing the Change in Health for an Additional Health Service

off, or even decline, until costs are associated with only small (if any) increases in health (point A). The state of "optimum health" is illustrated by point B, where the value of an additional increment to health equals the cost of producing that increment. CEA of health services applies this principle by comparing service A against a suitable alternative, such as "usual care" or no care (Garber et al. 1996). The first step of the CEA is to measure the additional health benefits of service A compared to the alternative, and also to measure the additional costs of producing those benefits. The second step is to compare these additional costs and health benefits (if any) as a C/E ratio.

One example of a cost-effectiveness evaluation of health services is the analysis performed by Mark and his associates (1995), who compared two treatments for patients with heart attacks. In simple terms, a major cause of a heart attack is a clogged coronary artery. When a blood clot, or thrombosis, forms in the artery, blood flow to the heart falls, which may cause a heart attack, or acute myocardial infarction. Several years ago, heart attack victims were treated with a clot-dissolving substance known as streptokinase. More recently, an alternative substance known as tissue plasminogen activator (or t-PA) became available. Mark and associates performed a CEA comparing use of t-PA with streptokinase based on data from 41,021 patients in Europe and the United States. One year following treatment, 10% of the patients treated with streptokinase died, while 9% of the patients treated with t-PA died. The 1% difference in mortality rates between the two groups was statistically significant, indicating that t-PA was more effective than streptokinase. Patients treated with t-PA, however, had higher costs ($2,216) than patients treated with streptokinase ($270), and t-PA's incremental cost-effectiveness ratio was $32,678 per year of life saved. The question that CEA cannot answer is whether the additional cost of treating heart attack patients with t-PA ($1,946 = $2,216 − $270 per patient) is worth the additional benefit (11 lives saved per 1,000 patients treated). Health professionals in the United States have answered "yes" to this question, and t-PA is now used widely for treating patients with acute myocardial infarction.

Although this example illustrates a CEA of *two* health services, CEA also may be used to compare the costs and benefits of *several* health services to guide resource allocation decisions (Patrick and Erickson 1993). Physicians, health maintenance organizations, state and federal health programs, and other decision makers often make daily decisions about how best to allocate scarce resources across a wide variety of health services to achieve the most health benefits. The decisions are difficult to make because the trade-offs between screening for breast cancer, immunizations, bypass surgery for coronary artery disease, and other health services are not obvious. Although CEA cannot decide how to allocate scarce resources across health services, it can identify the trade-offs by defining and comparing their costs and outcomes.

Comparing the costs and outcomes of different health services is easier if the outcomes are measured the same way for each service. In CEA of health services, a variety of outcome measures exist, such as the number of heart attacks prevented, disability days averted, years of life saved, or years of life gained (Torrance et al. 1996). Because years of life saved or gained are convenient and easily understood measures, they are widely used outcome measures for comparing different health services (Detsky and Redelmeier 1998; Gold, Siegel, et al. 1996; Graham et al. 1998; Tengs et al. 1995; Wright and Weinstein 1998).

To compare the cost and outcome trade-offs of health services, Tengs and her colleagues (1995) reported the cost-effectiveness of 587 "life-saving interventions" in the United States, each defined as a behavioral intervention and/or technology that reduces the probability of premature death in a target population, based on cost per year of life saved. The median medical intervention cost $19,000 per year of life saved, while the median injury reduction intervention cost $48,000 per year of life saved. Table 5.2 presents C/E ratios for selected

TABLE 5.2   Cost-Effectiveness Ratios for Selected Health Services

Service	Cost Per Year of Lives Saved
Immunization for all infants and preschool children (vs. scattered efforts)	≤$0
Influenza vaccination for all citizens	$140
Pneumonia vaccination for people age 65+	$1,800-$2,200
Pneumonia vaccination for low-risk people age 25-44	$66,000
Smoking cessation advice for men age 35-39	$1,400
Smoking cessation advice for women age 35-39	$2,900
Hypertension screening for asymptomatic men age 20	$48,000
Hypertension screening for asymptomatic men age 60	$11,000
Hypertension screening for asymptomatic women age 20	$87,000
Hypertension screening for asymptomatic women age 60	$17,000
Mammography every 3 years for women age 50-65	$2,700
Annual mammography for women age 55-64	$110,000
Left main coronary artery bypass graft surgery (vs. medical management)	$2,300-$5,600
Two-vessel coronary artery bypass graft surgery (vs. medical management)	$28,000-$75,000
Heart transplantation for patients age 55 or younger with favorable prognosis	$3,600
Heart transplantation for patients age 50 with terminal heart disease	$100,000
Home dialysis for chronic end-stage renal disease	$20,000-$23,000
Center dialysis for end-stage renal disease	$55,000-$64,000
Neonatal intensive care for low birth weight infants	$270,000

SOURCE: Adapted from "Five-Hundred Life-Saving Interventions and Their Cost-Effectiveness," Tengs et al. © Copyright 1995 by *Risk Analysis*.

preventive and therapeutic services. Although some preventive services, such as immunization for infants, are cost-saving, most services entail costs to save a year of life. An inspection of the table reveals that the cost per year of life saved depends on several factors, such as the prevalence of the disease in the target population (pneumonia and hypertension), gender (smoking cessation and hypertension screening), frequency of delivery (mammography), extent of the procedure (coronary artery bypass surgery), prognosis (heart transplantation), and site of treatment (dialysis treatment).

These and other C/E ratios presented by Tengs and her coauthors are valuable because they explicate the inherent trade-offs in allocating resources to one intervention rather than another. When a fixed budget must be allocated across health services for a given population, the goal is to allocate those limited funds in such a way as to produce the greatest amount of health (in this case, years of life saved) in the population. Just like the familiar tables comparing brands of merchandise in *Consumer Reports*, tables showing the ranking and C/E ratios of health services also convey which services are "best buys"—those that promote the greatest amount of health at the lowest cost (Russell et al. 1996). In some cases, the choices may be relatively simple, such as targeting older rather than younger men for hypertension screening because the C/E ratio declines with age (see Table 5.2). In other cases, the choices may be complex and difficult, such as deciding the relative allocations toward cost-effective preventive services versus such high-cost services as heart transplants for terminal patients and neonatal care for low birth weight infants. When resource allocation decisions are being made about identifiable lives that may be lost (such as neonatal care for low birth weight infants), society tends to favor allocating resources toward those lives rather than less dramatic and more cost-effective alternatives, such as prevention (Eisenberg 1989).

In some cases, additional information about the incidence and prevalence of a disease or condition in the population is critical in making allocation decisions. For example, the resource implications of providing neonatal intensive care to 10 versus 100 low birth weight infants are enormous. In other cases, decision makers may want to know more about the *quality* of the lives that are being saved. Although "years of life saved/gained" captures the *quantity* of life produced by health services, it does not measure the *quality* of improvement produced by those services. For example, although coronary artery bypass surgery may add years to life, physical or psychological impairment may follow surgery and lower the quality of the remaining years of life. In addition, because the goal of many health services is not primarily to save lives but to avert disability over the lifetime of an individual, outcome measures that combine quality with quantity are superior to measures of quantity alone (Gold, Patrick, et al. 1996). In response, measures that capture both the quantity (duration) and quality of life have emerged, such as quality-adjusted life years (QALYs), years of healthy life, well years, health-adjusted person years, quality-adjusted life expectancy, and health-adjusted life expectancy (Gold, Siegel, et al. 1996).

To illustrate the QALY measure, Edelson and his colleagues (1990) examined the cost-effectiveness of medications for hypertension for persons aged 35 to 64 with diastolic blood pressure of 95 mm Hg or greater and no known coronary artery disease. For persons taking propranolol hydrochloride for 20 years, the cost per year of life saved was $10,900. Citing evidence that propranolol impairs quality of life more than captopril, another hypertensive medication, they assumed that each year of life while taking propranolol was worth 0.995 years without it, yielding a C/E ratio of $16,500 per QALY. In other words, if a person takes propranolol for 20 years, the side effects of the drug will reduce the quality of those years. Adjusting for the impairment to quality of life reduces the medication's benefit (or effect), and with a smaller denominator in the C/E ratio, the cost per unit of benefit (QALY) is greater.

STEPS IN CONDUCTING A COST-EFFECTIVENESS ANALYSIS

Drawing from Warner and Luce (1982), CEA consists of 11 basic steps that traverse a similar course as Acts I, II, and III of the evaluation process. In this section, each step of the CEA is summarized, and key methodological issues are reviewed. In practice, CEA is a much more complex undertaking than described here, with detailed methodological standards for performing each step (Gold, Patrick, et al. 1996; Haddix et al. 1996; Siegel, Weinstein, Russell, et al. 1996; Siegel, Weinstein, and Torrance 1996).

Steps 1-4: Organizing the CEA

The decision to conduct an evaluation in Act I of the evaluation process entails four basic steps:

1. Define the problem and objectives.
2. Identify alternatives.
3. Describe production relationships, or the CEA's conceptual model.
4. Define the perspective of the CEA.

Together, the four steps organize the evaluation in the following manner.

Defining the problem and the objective(s) entails developing an in-depth understanding of the problem, the program developed to address it, and the key outcome(s) that the program will produce to reduce or solve the problem. For example, in the CEA of pregnant smokers reviewed in Table 5.1, the problem is the harmful effects of smoking on the mother's and the baby's health during pregnancy. The program is a self-help smoking cessation booklet designed especially for pregnant smokers, and the outcome is whether the pregnant smoker quits smoking. To provide an example for health services, a major problem is mortality and morbidity from heart attacks (myocardial infarction). Coronary artery bypass graft surgery is a service that is expected to reduce the problem, and the outcome of the intervention is years of life saved.

Identifying alternatives is the next step and is a critical element of the evaluation. The core feature of a CEA is to compare an intervention with one or more alternatives. To answer the question "Is the program or service cost-effective?", you must first answer the question "Cost-effective compared to what?" (Banta and Luce 1983). The answer is critical because the choice of the alternative(s) will frame the results of the CEA. For any given program or health service, several alternatives will likely be possible, depending on the intervention, such as no action (immunization vs. no immunization), usual care (the *Pregnant Woman's Guide* vs. standard information), a less intensive or costly version of the same program (the *Pregnant Woman's Guide* vs. the American Lung Association manual), a different medium for delivering the intervention (such as self-help booklet vs. videocassette), surgery versus medical management, a medication vs. a placebo medication, and so forth.

Describing the production relationships follows. Here the goal is to develop a model that identifies all the resources required by the program or service as well as explaining how they work together to produce expected outcomes. A key aspect of the model is understanding the efficiency of the production process: What *kinds* of inputs are required, what is the proper *amount* of each input, and what *combination* of inputs produces the most outputs? A model describing the production process for each alternative serves as a framework for estimating their costs and benefits in later steps.

Models describing the conversion of program inputs into outputs can be either simple or complex. Simple models contain basic information about program inputs—for example, equipment, the specific types and amounts of labor, the number and types of activities performed, and so forth. Complex models employ linear programming, decision analysis, or other techniques to quantify production relationships between inputs and outputs. For example, Veney and Kaluzny (1998) used operations research methods to develop a model defining the relationships between inputs and the number of clients served by a clinic. The conversion of inputs into outputs is often a "black box" of health programs, and regardless of the method chosen, the goal is to improve the visibility and knowledge of how this conversion process actually works.

Defining the perspective, or viewpoint, of the CEA is a critical fourth step. That is, the costs and effects of a CEA might be different from the point of view of society, the organization paying for the program, the person receiving the program or service, the provider, or other groups (Eisenberg 1989; Russell et al. 1996). One way to choose the perspective of the CEA is to ask the question "Who is affected by the program?" (Russell et al. 1996). That is, who pays for the program, in terms of both monetary and nonmonetary costs? Is it an employer, a health insurance plan, a person, society at large, or another group? Who benefits from the program? Just those who receive it? Or do people who do not directly receive the program also benefit from it? What about the program's side effects? Are they borne by the program's participants or by others?

If the answers to these questions suggest that the costs, outcomes, and side effects of a program are distributed broadly across groups, CEA typically adopts a "societal" perspective, where everyone affected by the program is included in the analysis, as well as all the important outcomes and costs that flow from it, regardless of who experiences those outcomes and costs (Davidoff and Powe 1996; Russell et al. 1996). In contrast, a CEA conducted from a more narrow perspective might omit some outcomes and costs that are not relevant to that person or group. For example, if an employer is paying for a smoking cessation program for its employees, the CEA might consider only the costs and outcomes that directly affect the employer, such as the dollar cost of implementing the program and the impact of the program on employee productivity and medical expenses.

The perspective of the CEA may have a great influence on the analysis and its results. Although many analysts argue that the societal perspective is the proper one, an alternative approach is to conduct the CEA from more than one perspective and compare the results to see if they are similar or different (Eisenberg 1989). If the results are similar, the resource allocation decision may be straightforward. If the results are different across perspectives, the trade-offs between viewpoints become explicit, which may generate conflict in resource allocation decisions in Act III of the evaluation process.

In summary, Steps 1-4 essentially cover the same territory as Act I of the evaluation process, but they are customized to organize the evaluation to answer questions about the cost-effectiveness of a health program or service. In Step 5, the CEA moves into Act II of the evaluation process, where the CEA is actually conducted and the questions are answered.

Step 5: Identify, Measure, and Value Costs

The first, essential piece of information to conduct a CEA is the cost of the health program or service, which is the value of all resources used by the program or service. The identification of costs is guided by the perspective of the CEA in Step 4, which influences what costs are included and excluded in the analysis. Given one or more perspectives, the goal of Step 4 is to identify, measure, and value the costs of the health program or service, which may be divided into the following four basic types (Luce et al. 1996; Weinstein and Stason 1977).

Direct costs include all the goods, services, and other resources used to deliver the intervention, which may be divided into two groups, *intervention costs* and *nonintervention costs* (Eisenberg 1989; Luce et al. 1996). Intervention costs include all resources that are used in the delivery of the intervention, such as the cost of personnel, supplies, equipment, facilities, drugs, diagnostic tests, and other medical or nonmedical expenses. Nonintervention costs are resource costs that are part of the intervention but are borne by others. Examples include child care costs for a parent attending a smoking cessation program, travel costs to attend the program, or volunteer time spent caring for a sick child. Direct costs also include patient time costs, such as the time spent searching for a provider, traveling to the provider's clinic, and waiting in the office, as well as the time receiving treatment.

The second type of costs consists of *indirect* or *productivity* costs, which occur when there is lost or impaired ability to work or engage in leisure activities as a direct result of the intervention. These costs are often captured by the patient's time for recuperation and convalescence resulting from the intervention. If the outcome measure of the CEA is quality-adjusted life years, the morbidity costs may be measured in dollars and captured in the numerator of the C/E ratio, or they may be included in the assessment of QALYs due to the intervention and be captured in the denominator of the C/E ratio (Luce et al. 1996).

The third type are actual *cost savings* that occur from the prevention or alleviation of disease. As mentioned earlier, very few health programs and services are cost-saving, so this category is typically zero in most cost-effectiveness analyses.

The fourth type is *future costs*, which include the costs of disease that are unrelated to the intervention. For example, a person may participate in an exercise program, which may prevent a heart attack and premature death. By living longer, however, the person likely will require treatment for other diseases. Whether or not the future cost for treatment of later medical conditions should be included in a CEA is controversial. For example, if an exercise program successfully reduces heart attacks, decision makers may have little interest in whether program participants have another serious illness later in life. If these costs are small relative to the size of the C/E ratio, they can be safely ignored. If they are large, the C/E ratio should be calculated with and without them to determine their influence on the study's findings.

Step 6: Identify and Measure Effectiveness

The second piece of information essential to conducting a CEA is one or more estimates of the effectiveness, or benefits, of the health program or service. In general, benefits can be divided into two categories, *tangible* and *intangible*. Tangible benefits can be divided into four groups (Warner and Luce 1982). The first group consists of health care resource savings, or *economic benefits*, such as days of work loss avoided or the number of physician hours or days of hospital bed occupancy saved. The second group is composed of *intermediate outcomes*, such as the number of smokers who quit smoking in a smoking cessation program or the accuracy of a new diagnostic test compared to the standard test. The third group consists of final outcomes, or *personal health benefits*, such as years of life saved or QALYs, which have three components (Weinstein and Stason 1977):

1. the change in life expectancy (years of life saved) due to the intervention, relative to an alternative;
2. the change or improvement in quality of life due to the alleviation or prevention of morbidity, relative to an alternative; and
3. the change or decline in quality of life due to side effects of the intervention, relative to an alternative.

The fourth group consists of *social benefits*. That is, some health programs generate benefits for the people who participate in them as well as for society as a whole. For example, although the Medicare and Medicaid programs are designed to improve the health of their enrollees (a personal health benefit), they also generate social benefits by increasing access to health care in our society. Intangible benefits include the alleviation of pain and suffering from a medical condition, the relief from worry and stress for the individual and the individual's family, and other, similar kinds of benefits.

Most CEAs do not quantitatively measure all these benefits but instead focus on a relatively small but important set of them that, depending on the perspective of the CEA, are most relevant to a health program or service. For example, a CEA conducted from a societal perspective might take a very broad approach to the allocation of health resources and include all tangible and intangible benefits associated with the program or service. In contrast, a CEA conducted from the perspective of the organization implementing the program or service might have a more narrow focus and consider only those benefits that are important to the organization, such as intermediate outcomes and economic benefits. Because intangible benefits usually are difficult to measure quantitatively, regardless of the CEA's perspective, they often are not measured explicitly in CEAs. As mentioned earlier, if the outcome measure of the CEA is QALYs, the intangible benefits may be measured as part of the QALY (Eisenberg 1989).

Measures of a health program's or service's benefits are obtained by either conducting an impact evaluation or abstracting them from the literature. If estimates of an intervention's effectiveness are available from published studies, the evidence should be reviewed critically before going forward with the CEA. Two important issues are *quality* and *relevance*, or the internal and external validity of the studies (Drummond et al. 1997). In general, the greater the internal validity of the study, the greater the quality of the evidence. Similarly, the greater the similarity between the context of the published study and the proposed CEA, the greater the relevance, or external validity, of the prior work.

Step 7: Discount Future Costs and Effectiveness

If a program's costs and effects occur in a single year, the CEA proceeds to Step 8. If the costs and effects occur over several years, both must be "discounted" to their present value (Banta and Luce 1983; Warner and Luce 1982). For example, let's suppose that a program's costs and benefits occur over 5 years and that the cost of the program in each year is $100. On the one hand, we could simply add the costs of the program over 5 years to obtain a total program cost of $500 (5 × $100 = $500). The problem with this approach is that a dollar today is not worth the same amount as a dollar one or more years from now. That is, if people were asked whether they wanted a $100 today or 1 year from now, most people would place a higher value, or worth, on having the money today, which gives them the option of either spending or saving it. If they decided to save it for 1 year at 5% interest, the $100 would be worth $105 dollars at the end of 1 year. Discounting is the reverse process: The $105 a year from now has a present value of $100 at the 5% discount rate. In short, discounting is a way of standardizing the worth of dollars spent over a number of years to make them commensurate with current dollars.

TABLE 5.3   Discounting the Stream of Dollar Costs for a 5-Year Program

Future Year	Undiscounted Costs	Discount Factor	Discounted Costs
0	$100.00	$1/(1 + .05)^0$	$100.00
1	100.00	$1/(1 + .05)^1$	95.24
2	100.00	$1/(1 + .05)^2$	90.70
3	100.00	$1/(1 + .05)^3$	86.38
4	100.00	$1/(1 + .05)^4$	82.27
Total	$500.00		454.59

Table 5.3 illustrates undiscounted and discounted costs for a 5-year program. The undiscounted costs of the program are $500. The formula for the annual discount factor is $1/(1 + r)^n$, where r is the discount rate and n refers to the number of years from now. Today, discount rates of 3% are recommended (Lipscomb et al. 1996), although rates of 5% or 6% are often used (Eisenberg 1989). When a 5% discount rate is applied, the undiscounted dollar costs are $500, and the discounted costs are $454.59. The sum of the discounted stream of future costs is known as the *present value* of the future costs.

Discounting is a separate concept from inflation, which captures fluctuations in market prices of goods and services. Inflation typically is addressed by deflating dollars to their value in a single year *before* discounting is performed (Warner and Luce 1982). Discounting effectiveness, such as years of life saved, is controversial, because many people believe that a year of life saved today has the same worth as a year of life saved in any future year; however, discounting of effectiveness typically is performed in CEAs. Weinstein and Stason (1977) and Lipscomb et al. (1996) explain the reason for discounting effectiveness through the following example. Assume that a program costs $100 per year, and that spending $100 saves 10 lives (or 1 life per $10 spent). If the $100 were invested at a 10% rate of return, in 1 year it would be worth $110, and with the $110, it would be possible to save 11 lives. If the initial $100 was invested for 2 years, it would be worth $121, and 12 lives could be saved. Thus, the longer the program is delayed (by investing the money rather than implementing the program), the more dollars there are to save more lives, creating an incentive to defer the program forever. In addition, if the aim of the C/E ratio is to compare costs and effects, the intervention's streams of costs and effects over time should be measured in a similar manner. Therefore, if the C/E ratio is composed of dollars discounted to their present value, then discounting effectiveness also is methodologically sound because it leads to a consistent comparison of costs and effectiveness in the ratio (Lipscomb et al. 1996).

In summary, discounting is a method of converting costs and benefits over time into their respective present values. Programs that spend money early to achieve benefits further downstream are less likely to be cost-effective. Because preventive health services treat people who may never become ill, these programs are at a disadvantage under CEA (Emery and Schneiderman 1989). In addition, CEA and discounting also work against the elderly. Because the young have longer remaining life spans than older adults, life-saving interventions by definition produce more years of life for young people than old people. Thus, programs for older adults are at a disadvantage when compared to programs for the young.

Step 8: Sensitivity Analysis

Uncertainty exists in all CEAs, and a large number of assumptions inevitably are made to deal with them. A major issue in CEA is whether these assumptions have influenced the results of the evaluation. Sensitivity analysis is a systematic approach for determining whether a CEA yields the same results if different assumptions are made.

For example, a CEA is conducted with a 5% discount rate. Is this the "right" rate to use? Would the results be the same if different discount rates were used? Lipscomb et al. (1996) recommend that sensitivity analyses of discount rates use a range from 0% to 7%. The lower bound (0%) indicates the results of the CEA without discounting. The upper bound represents a ceiling for interest rates in current markets.

Similar exercises can be conducted using other parameters of a CEA. In Table 5.1, for example, 14% of the pregnant smokers who received the *Pregnant Woman's Guide* quit smoking. Would the cost-effectiveness of the program change if the quit rate was 7%? Would it change if it was 21%? Would the results change if the costs of staff time to run the program were valued differently? Or would the results change if the booklets cost twice as much to develop and print?

In short, a sensitivity analysis alters key values in the CEA to find out whether their different levels alter the main conclusions of the study. This entails three basic steps:

1. Identify the parameters that are most uncertain in the analysis (such as the estimates of program effectiveness or the discount rate).
2. Specify the possible range over which these parameters may vary.
3. Calculate C/E ratios based on different combinations of the parameters that represent the best guess, most conservative, and least conservative estimates. (Drummond et al. 1997)

For example, Hatziandreu et al. (1995) performed these steps in their CEA of three programs to increase use of bicycle helmets and decrease head injuries among children. They examined whether the results changed if different assumptions were made about the percentage of children wearing helmets, the percentage of children who were injured, the percentage of injured children who were hospitalized, the price of the helmets, the risk of head injury for a cyclist not wearing a helmet, and other factors. They found that the basic results of the CEA were relatively stable under these different conditions.

Step 9: Address Equity Issues

Many public health programs are designed to benefit certain population groups in society. For example, Medicare was created to improve access to care for older adults, and Medicaid was created to achieve the same goal for low-income people. An obvious objective of a CEA of these programs is to determine whether the programs in fact have increased access in their respective target groups. More specifically, equity issues are concerned about the *distribution* of benefits across groups. For example, did the health outcomes of CEA reflect small improvements for a large number of people or large improvements for a few (Siegel et al. 1996b)?

A related question is whether similar results are obtained for different gender, racial, or other subgroups. For example, Joyce et al. (1988) compared the cost-effectiveness of government programs for low-income people in reducing neonatal mortality or death in the first 27 days of life across different racial groups. The CEA examined the following programs: teenage family planning use; the supplemental food program for women, infants, and children (WIC); use of community health centers and maternal and infant care projects; abortion; prenatal care; and neonatal intensive care. They found that early initiation of prenatal care was most cost-effective in reducing neonatal mortality for blacks and whites, and that blacks benefit more per dollar invested than whites. At the other extreme, neonatal intensive care, which is the most effective means of reducing neonatal mortality rates, was one of the least cost-effective for both racial groups.

Less obvious equity issues might arise in the calculation of the C/E ratios (Warner and Luce 1982). For example, the calculation of program costs might include the value of a person's time, and wage rates may be used to measure those costs. But what wage rate should be used in the analysis? Wages for men and women differ, and they also vary by racial and ethnic group, as well as for working and retired people. Do the distribution of program costs and the results of the analysis change when different assumptions about wage rates are applied? These are important issues, particularly for CEAs conducted from a societal perspective, and sensitivity analysis is a useful tool for examining their influence on the evaluation's conclusions.

Steps 10 and 11: Use of CEA Results in Decision Making

After the CEA is completed at the end of Act II, the evaluation process moves into Act III, where the results are disseminated to decision makers, who may or may not use the findings in their resource allocation decisions. One method of disseminating results is to publish them, and Siegel and colleagues (Siegel, Weinstein, Russell, et al. 1996; Siegel, Weinstein, and Torrance 1996) have developed guidelines for presenting CEA findings in journal articles and technical reports. Lengthy reports, however, may be less accessible to decision makers, who typically prefer shorter, concise forms of oral and written presentation of evaluation results. Mechanisms for encouraging the use of evaluation results in decision making are addressed in more detail in Chapter 10.

SUMMARY

In summary, CEA has become a highly visible form of evaluation in the health program literature, and CEA studies of health services have increased considerably over the past three decades. CEA is a flexible set of tools that are grounded in economic theory and designed to aid decision making. The results of a CEA, however, do *not* make decisions about resource allocation, for they always involve judgments of program worth, which can be made only by decision makers. The terms *cost-effective* and *cost-saving* have different meanings and are often confused. Although many health programs and services produce benefits that are deemed to be worth their cost (or are "cost-effective"), relatively few of them bring in more resources than they cost (or are "cost-saving").

In Act I of the evaluation process, decision makers pose questions that are answered by conducting an impact evaluation, a CEA, an evaluation of program implementation (or process evaluation), or some combination of the three types of evaluation. Methods of evaluating program implementation, either as the sole purpose of the evaluation or together with an impact evaluation or CEA, are reviewed in the next chapter.

LIST OF TERMS

Benefits (effects)

Cost-saving

Cost-benefit analysis (CBA)

Cost-effectiveness analysis (CEA)

Cost-effectiveness ratio (C/E ratio)

Cost-minimization analysis (CMA)

Cost-utility analysis (CUA)

Costs

Direct costs

Discounting

Economic benefits

Equity issues

Future costs

Indirect (productivity) costs

Intangible benefits

Intermediate outcomes

Intervention costs

Nonintervention costs

Personal health benefits

Perspective

Present value

Quality-adjusted life
  years (QALYs)

Relative efficiency

Sensitivity analysis

Social benefits

Tangible benefits

STUDY QUESTIONS

1. Can a cost-effectiveness analysis be conducted if the program's effects are unknown? Should a cost-effectiveness analysis be conducted if the program has no effect? What are the two basic forms of cost-effectiveness analysis in the health field?

2. What is the difference between average vs. incremental cost-effectiveness?

3. What are the basic steps in conducting a cost-effectiveness analysis?

4. Why is the perspective of the cost-effectiveness evaluation important? What is meant by discounting and sensitivity analysis? Why do we do them?

5. Do the results of a cost-effectiveness analysis make decisions about the program?

6. Does "cost-effectiveness" mean the same thing as "cost-saving"?

CHAPTER 6

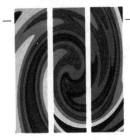

Evaluation of Program Implementation

I f one or more questions are asked about the implementation of a program in Act I of the evaluation process, the next step is to design an evaluation that yields answers for each question. Designing an evaluation of a program's implementation can be more challenging than designing an impact evaluation, mainly because impact evaluations have a more limited scope. In most impact evaluations, questions are asked about the outcomes produced by the program, and the sole purpose is to estimate program impacts. As described in Chapter 4, designing an impact evaluation entails choosing, from a "menu" of standard designs, one impact design that best fits the program and that has the greatest internal and external validity. In short, the narrow scope and the well-defined, alternative designs provide a *structure* for organizing and conducting the impact evaluation, which produces a quantitative estimate of program impacts.

This structured, menu-driven approach does not apply to implementation evaluations, mainly because they have a broader scope. Many different questions can be asked about the implementation of a program, and different implementation designs may be required to answer each one, using either quantitative or qualitative information, or both. In most cases, the design of an implementation evaluation must be *customized*, or created from scratch, to answer the *specific* questions that are asked about a *specific* program. The tighter the connection between the questions about a program and the methods for answering them, the more rigorous and structured the evaluation will be. Thus, to design an implementation evaluation, the evaluator must *develop* a structure, or framework, to guide the evaluation by clearly specifying

1. the questions that are asked about the implementation of a program,
2. the evaluation designs for answering them,
3. the quantitative and qualitative information that will be collected for each question, and
4. how the information will be analyzed to answer each question.

The purpose of this chapter is to describe basic approaches to designing an implementation evaluation. Because questions drive the design of implementation evaluations, different *types* of questions may suggest different *designs* for answering them. In the next section, different designs are presented for evaluating program implementation. In the second section, different types of implementation questions are presented, and one or more designs for answering them are described. A final section summarizes methodological issues that must be addressed in answering all types of questions about program implementation.

TYPES OF EVALUATION DESIGNS FOR ANSWERING IMPLEMENTATION QUESTIONS

Designs for answering implementation questions have two dimensions: the *purpose* of the design and the *timing* of data collection (Aday 1996; Gehlbach 1993; Miller 1991; Patton 1997). One purpose of implementation designs is simply to *describe* events, activities, or behavior that occurred in a health program, often with the goal of creating a "profile" of "what went on" in the program. A second purpose of implementation designs is to *explain* events, activities, or behavior that occurred in a health program, typically with the goal of improving understanding of them. Comparison is the basic strategy of explanatory designs. For example, if a subset of participants regularly miss scheduled program events, the characteristics of participants who attend and do not attend the events can be compared, and differences between the two groups may provide insights that at least partly explain the absenteeism.

Implementation designs also may differ based on the timing of data collection. In a *cross-sectional* design, data about program events, activities, behaviors, attitudes, or other factors are collected at *one* point in time. In a *longitudi-*

TABLE 6.1   Typology of Implementation Evaluation Designs

Timing of Data Collection	Purpose of the Design	
	Descriptive	Explanatory
Cross-Sectional	A ✓ Describe program events, activities, or behavior at one point in time	C Compare program events, activities, or behavior at one point in time
Longitudinal	B Describe program events, activities, or behavior at two or more points in time	D Compare events, activities, or behavior at two or more points in time

nal design, data about the program are collected at *two or more* points in time. In longitudinal designs, the usual goal is to track changes in these factors over time, and therefore the same data are collected at each point in time.

The purpose and timing dimensions can be combined to create four basic types of implementation designs, as shown in Table 6.1. The goal of the descriptive cross-sectional designs (cell A) is simply to describe the program at a single point in time. For example, if a health clinic is implemented in a high school (Borenstein et al. 1996; Walter et al. 1996), a random sample of students may be surveyed to find out if they are satisfied with the clinic. The goal of descriptive longitudinal designs (cell B) is to describe the program at two or more points in time. For example, annual surveys of students may be conducted each school year to describe trends in student satisfaction over time.

The goal of explanatory cross-sectional designs (cell C) is to understand or explain what is happening in the program at a single point in time. For example, the characteristics of students who are satisfied and dissatisfied with the high school clinic can be compared to understand why satisfaction varies across students. In explanatory longitudinal designs (cell D), the goal is to understand how the program is changing over two or more points in time. For example, if annual surveys of students are conducted, the characteristics of students who are dissatisfied can be compared over time to find out if these characteristics are consistent or vary from year to year.

The four basic designs apply to both quantitative and qualitative methods of data collection and analysis. Quantitative information—whether from surveys of high school students, program administrative records, medical charts, or other sources—is collected and analyzed in virtually all implementation evaluations using one or more of the four designs. Simple descriptive statistics may be all that is necessary to describe the characteristics and features of programs and their participants. In explanatory designs, bivariate statistical techniques—and sometimes multivariable analysis of the data—are performed to compare one aspect of the program with another.

Qualitative information also can be collected through one or more of the designs. In general, evaluations collect qualitative information because it can improve knowledge and understanding of what happened in the program in the following ways (Maxwell 1998):

▶ Understanding the *meaning*, for program participants, of the events, personal encounters, and situations they experienced in the program. This application is useful particularly when programs have participants from different cultures who may experience the same intervention in different ways.

▶ Understanding the *context* of the program and the influence of this context on participant behavior.

▶ Identifying *unintended consequences* of the program.

▶ Understanding the *processes* that lead to observed outcomes of the program, and why observed and expected outcomes might be different.

▶ Generating new *causal explanations* of why the program did or did not work, which may lead to revisions of a program's theory of cause and effect or theory of implementation.

In short, qualitative information complements quantitative information; both are essential for understanding program performance.

Different qualitative methods exist, such as case studies, content analysis, ethnography, focus groups, informal interviewing, and participant and nonparticipant observation. Qualitative methods can be applied in all four designs of Table 6.1. For example, a qualitative analysis of "deviant cases," or students who are highly satisfied and highly dissatisfied with the high school clinic, could be conducted (Weiss 1998a). Using a descriptive design, focus groups of these students could be conducted to build an in-depth understanding of what students do and do not like about the high school clinic and the reasons why (cell A in Table 6.1). Then, an explanatory design could be used to compare how these views vary from year to year and why (cells B and D in Table 6.1; Dean 1994).

TYPES OF QUESTIONS AND DESIGNS
FOR ANSWERING THEM

The four types of designs can be applied to answer a wide variety of questions about the implementation of a health program. In general, questions about program implementation can be divided into two broad groups: questions posed to monitor implementation, ultimately to help administrators manage the program, and questions asked to explain the program outcomes that were estimated in an impact evaluation. In this section, each group of questions and the designs for answering them are reviewed.

*implem.
outcomes.*

Monitoring Program Implementation

The first category consists of questions asked to find out "what's going on" in the program by *monitoring* the activities, events, behavior, or other relevant phenomena of the program (Rossi et al. 1999; Scheirer 1994; Veney and Kaluzny 1998). A major purpose of monitoring is to provide information to administrators about the program's progress in achieving objectives on a regular basis, information that can be used to improve program performance (Scheirer 1994). Although monitoring is important for programs of all sizes, it is essential in large, complex programs that are difficult to manage in the field. As the size and complexity of programs increase, so does the need for management information systems to help administrators monitor and manage their implementation.

Common questions for monitoring health programs that deliver services to people are listed in Table 6.2 on the left. The right column presents samples of each question from the Medicare demonstration, which delivered a package of preventive services to 1,250 older adults in the intervention group (see Chapter 3).

Most of these questions can be answered using descriptive study designs and data collected at one or several points in time (cells A and B in Table 6.1). Only the fourth question requires an explanatory design for comparing the health risks and personal characteristics of adults with the services they received.

TABLE 6.2   Common Questions for Monitoring Programs That Deliver Services

Questions for Monitoring Program Services	Sample Questions for the Medicare Demonstration
1. Who is the program serving?	1. What are the personal characteristics and health risks of older adults in the program?
2. What services were provided?	2. What mix of health promotion and disease prevention services did adults in the program receive?
3. Who receives what kind of services?	3. What are the personal characteristics of the older adults who received each service?
4. Are the services appropriate?	4. Are health risks and personal characteristics associated properly with the services that adults received?
5. Are people satisfied with the services?	5. Are older adults satisfied with the services they received?
6. What outcomes did people experience?	6. Did older adults in the program change their self-efficacy, health behavior, and utilization of health services? Did their health status change?

Monitoring also can be linked to a program's hierarchy of objectives. For example, the immediate, intermediate, and ultimate objectives of the Medicare prevention program were presented in Table 3.4. Immediate objectives consisted of recruiting clinics, providers, and Medicare enrollees into the program; intermediate objectives focused on the delivery of the preventive services to older adults; and ultimate objectives were expected changes in health status and health care utilization and costs. Because intermediate objectives can be attained only if immediate objectives are achieved, and ultimate objectives can be attained only if intermediate objectives are achieved, monitoring progress throughout the hierarchy is a useful strategy for identifying and correcting implementation problems.

Clearly, a seemingly infinite number of monitoring questions can be asked about a program. For example, Shortell (1984) suggests comparing projected and actual performance, such as discrepancies between projected and actual client enrollment, delays in moving from one phase to the next phase of a program, and other markers such as turnover of key personnel, number of staff meetings canceled, and other signals of potential performance problems. Similarly, Affholter (1994) recommends monitoring program outcomes to keep managers apprised of performance and focus attention on improving results.

Because so many aspects of a program can be tracked, monitoring systems can become unwieldy and therefore have less value. This problem can be avoided by asking questions in Act I of the evaluation process that target key areas of the program, then monitoring those areas over time. For example, Figure 3.4 presented the major steps of implementing New York City's lead poisoning screening program. To monitor progress, an information system was developed for monitoring the following activities over time, which documented progress in achieving the major steps (President and Fellows of Harvard College 1975):

▶ Blood tests administered

▶ Cases of lead poisoning detected

▶ Recurrent cases of lead poisoning

▶ Housing units inspected

▶ Housing units found hazardous

▶ Housing units repaired

These types of monitoring are very similar to continuous quality improvement (CQI) techniques that are common in business and industry (Colton 1997). Originally developed in the manufacturing sector, CQI is an evaluation approach that is relatively common in health and human service organizations. A central feature of CQI is the continuous monitoring of service delivery processes to correct variation from the desired level of performance. In service delivery organizations, CQI typically consists of the following components (Colton 1997):

▶ Identify processes of service delivery by developing flowcharts illustrating the steps for delivering services and their connections.

▶ Determine client satisfaction with the steps in the process.

▶ Collect data indicating the level and intensity of service delivery, particularly in areas where clients are dissatisfied (for example, client waiting times at an admission site).

▶ Determine thresholds of acceptable variation (for example, determine the lower and upper limits of acceptable client waiting times at an admission site).

▶ Correct the process to reduce variation (for example, if waiting times exceed an upper threshold, the admission process is examined to identify potential causes, which are targeted for correction).

▶ Assess the effectiveness of the corrections through continued monitoring to determine whether variation was reduced (for example, tracking the percentage of client waiting times that are still above the threshold).

▶ Continue to monitor and correct as required.

In short, CQI is a technique for evaluating work flow processes in the delivery of health services and may apply when the evaluation questions from Act I address this topic.

Explaining Program Outcomes

The second group of questions consists of those asked to explain the observed outcomes of the program. Impact evaluations provide information about whether a program achieved its objectives. In general, impact evaluations yield one or more of the following three basic answers: the program worked, the program did not work, or the program had unintended consequences. Although decision makers want to know about program impacts, they also want to know *why* those impacts were obtained. This is because information about program impacts alone offers little guidance to decision makers about how to fix programs that do not work, how to identify and replicate successful elements of a program in other settings, or how to avoid unintended consequences of a program in the future. A *comprehensive* evaluation of a health program includes an evaluation of program impacts and implementation, where program implementation is examined to explain program impacts.

Questions asked to explain program impacts may be divided into the following groups:

1. Questions about why the program had no effects
2. Questions about why the program had beneficial effects
3. Questions about why the program had unintended consequences

Each group of questions and designs for answering them are reviewed in this section.

Questions About Why the Program Worked

When an impact evaluation reveals that a health program has beneficial results, the next logical question is often "What worked?" (King et al. 1987; Patton 1990, 1997). One strategy for answering this question is to identify people in the treatment group who showed the *greatest* and *least* amount of change, an exploratory design known as "disaggregating" (Weiss 1998a). For example, in the Medicare demonstration, the package of preventive services reduced dietary fat intake among older adults, where dietary fat is measured by percentage of calories from fat. At the 2-year follow-up, two groups can be identified among adults in the treatment group who consumed too much fat: those who decreased their dietary fat the most and those who increased their dietary fat the most. An explanatory design can be used to compare the characteristics of the two groups to determine whether other factors may have influenced the different outcomes. An explanatory design also can be used to determine whether the mix of preventive services in the group that decreased its dietary fat was significantly different from the mix of services in the group that increased its dietary fat. If a significant difference in the mix of services is obtained, it may also explain why the two groups changed in opposite directions. In addition, qualitative methods of data collection, such as focus groups composed of adults from the two groups, may provide insights about why some people changed and others did not.

Questions About Why the Program Did Not Work

Programs may not work for one or more reasons, which may be independent or work in combination. The following list of questions is a "checklist" for systematically reviewing alternative explanations of faulty program performance.

Was the program implemented as intended? Impact evaluations of health programs either explicitly or implicitly assume that the program was implemented as intended. This may or may not be the case. If an impact evaluation indicates that a health program does not work, it may be because the program was never implemented, was implemented but never reached expected levels of implementation, or was implemented in a different manner than intended (Gottfredson et al. 1998; Scheirer 1994).

The classic example of this problem in the evaluation literature is Pressman and Wildavsky's (1984) implementation study of a $23 million federal economic development program to increase employment of minority groups in Oakland, California. In 1969, 3 years after the program began, only $3 million had been spent, and very little had been accomplished in terms of minority employment. No obvious explanations accounted for the low performance levels. Congress had appropriated the funds, city officials and employers approved the program, and there was widespread agreement and little conflict. Instead, the implementation problems were of an "everyday character." As described in Chapter 3, program implementation may be viewed as a "chain of events": A must occur before B, B before C, and so forth, until the outcome at the end of the chain is reached. The more links in the chain, and the more connections among the links, the more complex implementation becomes. In Oakland, the chain had many links, numerous approvals and clearances from many officials were required to move from link to link, and agreements had to be maintained after they were reached, which made it very difficult to make ordinary events happen. Rather than thinking implementation is easy, Pressman and Wildavsky concluded that program implementation, under the best of circumstances, is often difficult to accomplish.

Descriptive designs that monitor program implementation, as described earlier, can provide useful information for determining whether each phase of a program was completed as planned. Tracking a program's progress through its hierarchy of objectives is a reasonable way of judging whether the program was actually implemented as intended. Alternatively, if a program's theory of implementation is defined in Act I of the evaluation process, its "chain of events" also can be used to verify whether the program was implemented as intended. For example, in the lead poisoning program's theory of implementation illustrated in Figure 3.4, the program was supposed to screen thousands of children in the community for lead poisoning, treat children with high lead blood levels, and repair lead-contaminated housing. If one or more of these activities is not accomplished, evidence exists that the program was not implemented as intended, at least in part.

Was the intervention strong enough to make a difference? This question raises two concerns. First, if everyone in the treatment group actually receives the program, the intervention itself may not be strong enough to cause a difference, relative to the control group (Chen and Rossi 1983). For example, heavy smoking is an addictive behavior that is difficult to change. In the population of heavy smokers, smoking cessation programs that simply provide smokers with information about the harmful consequences of smoking are often too weak to change behavior. In essence, there is a problem with the program's the-ory of cause and effect, where the program is insufficient to cause intended be-havior change. To examine this issue, for example, the smokers who partici-pated in the program can be interviewed in depth to collect detailed information about their perceptions of the program and why it had little influ-ence on their behavior. This information can be obtained through a descriptive design using qualitative methods of data collection.

The second concern is that even though a program is implemented as in-tended, exposure to the program often varies across members of the treatment group. This situation may result in a "dose-response" relationship, where the program has beneficial outcomes for those receiving all elements of the pro-gram but little or no benefits for those receiving part or none of the program (Rossi et al. 1999; Scheirer 1994). A descriptive design can be used to examine whether exposure to the program varied greatly among members of the treat-ment group. If the percentage of unexposed people is relatively large, explana-tory designs can be used to examine whether members who were exposed fully to the program had better outcomes than those who had incomplete or no ex-posure to the program.

For example, in the Medicare demonstration, older adults in the intervention group received an annual package of preventive services for 2 years at their doc-tors' offices. In the first year of the program, 90% of the adults in the treatment group received the intervention, and 83% of the adults received the interven-tion in the second year. Although exposure declined in the second year, more than 90% of the people in the treatment group had some exposure, suggesting that a "dose-response" effect might not be a critical factor influencing out-comes.

In contrast to these findings, Pentz and associates (1990) examined the im-pact of a multiple-component classroom program to reduce use of alcohol, cig-arettes, and marijuana in young teenagers. They found that program implemen-tation varied greatly among teachers delivering the intervention, and that a dose-response relationship existed in program outcomes. Based on self-reports, the percentage of students who smoked *decreased* from 15% to 14% among students exposed fully to the program. Among students partly exposed to the program, smoking *increased* from 13% to 20%. For students in the control group, the percentage of students smoking also *increased* from 13% to 24%. These results indicate that the program, when implemented fully, was effective in preventing an increase in smoking among young teens.

Finally, if a dose-response relationship is detected, the next logical question is to explain why some people had less exposure to the program than others (Scheirer 1994). Answers to this question will provide managers with information that may lead to program changes that improve exposure and, ultimately, program impacts.

Did program implementation follow established protocols? Impact evaluations normally assume that implementation is similar across settings; however, health programs often are implemented by different people in different organizations in different geographic areas. If implementation varies for members of the treatment group, statistical power and the strength of the intervention may be reduced, which reduce the likelihood of detecting a program impact (Rossi et al. 1999; also see Chapter 4). To illustrate this point, Lipsey (1997) conducted a meta-analysis of 76 evaluations of interventions with juvenile delinquents who had a history of violent or other serious offenses, and who were treated in institutional facilities. The two most important factors influencing outcomes were the type of treatment provided and the integrity of implementation, defined as how closely adherence to protocols was monitored and how fully the treatment was implemented as intended. As shown in Table 6.3, program effects were greatest when the integrity of implementation was the highest (0.29 to 0.62), and the effects were lowest—almost zero—when the integrity of implementation was lowest (0.02 to 0.30). Descriptive designs that monitor program implementation can collect information to determine whether protocols vary across settings. Both cross-sectional and longitudinal designs are relevant, because adherence to protocols may vary over the life of a program. According to Lipsey (1997), if the data are unavailable, simply knowing whether adherence to protocols was monitored may provide a minimum amount of information to assess the influence of this factor on program impacts.

Did the control group receive a similar intervention from another source? Impact evaluations assume that only the treatment group receives the program; however, the control group also may be inadvertently exposed to the program as well. To check whether "contamination" of the control group has occurred, an explanatory design can be used to compare exposure in the treatment and control groups. For example, in the Medicare demonstration, a major concern was whether older adults in the control group were receiving health promotion and disease prevention services from their health care providers, who also were delivering these services to adults in the treatment group (Patrick et al. 1999). To address this concern, at the end of the intervention, adults in the treatment and control groups were presented with an inventory of the key preventive services in the intervention and asked to indicate the services they had received from their providers. The exposure to the intervention's preventive services

TABLE 6.3   How Type of Treatment and Integrity of Implementation Influence the Outcome of Programs to Reduce Juvenile Delinquency

| | Integrity of Treatment Implementation | | |
	Low	Medium	High
Group I: Skills training Cognitive-behavioral Multiservice	0.29	0.45	0.62
Group II: Counseling Drug abuse Mileau therapy Community residential	0.20	0.37	0.53
Group III: Group counseling Challenge programs	0.07	0.24	0.40
Group IV: Employment-related Guided group Teaching family home	0.02	0.14	0.30

SOURCE: Adapted from Lipsey MW, "What Can You Build With Thousands of Bricks? Musings on the Cumulation of Knowledge." In: *New Directions for Evaluation* 1997; 76:21.

was much higher in the treatment than in the control group, indicating that contamination was less of a concern in this evaluation.

Did external events weaken the program's impact? Even though adults in the control group of the Medicare demonstration had significantly less exposure to preventive services from their health care providers, they may have been exposed to these services from other sources. For example, one of the disease prevention services was a flu immunization, and adults in the control group may have received a flu shot from another source in the community, such as the local health department's flu shot program. In this case, an external event, the health department's program, may have weakened the program's impact. Alternatively, a prominent person in society may develop a potentially fatal disease, sparking greater societal interest in preventive services and prompting increased preventive visits among members of the control group (with little or no effect on treatment group members, because they already are receiving a high level of preventive care). A longitudinal, descriptive design that systematically monitors the environment over the life of a program is required to detect external events that have the potential to weaken program impacts.

Did the program's theory of cause and effect work as expected? A program may have no impacts because the program's theory of cause and effect is faulty, the program's theory of implementation is faulty, or both have faults (see Chapter 3). If answers to the above questions reveal that the program was actually implemented as intended, the program may have no impacts because of faults with its theory of cause and effect. To examine this question, explanatory designs may be applied to determine whether the "causal chain" in the program's theory of cause and effect is working as expected.

For example, the theory of cause and effect of the Medicare demonstration is presented in Figure 3.1. The theory posits that the package of preventive services will increase the self-efficacy of older adults in performing preventive health behaviors—a "mediating" variable, which will increase healthy behavior and ultimately decrease decline in health status. To examine this causal chain, the self-efficacy of adults was measured at baseline for the following five health behaviors: alcohol consumption, dietary fat intake, exercise, smoking cessation, and weight control. At the end of the 2-year demonstration, the self-efficacy of treatment group adults in exercising regularly had increased, while the exercise efficacy beliefs of the control group had declined. No differences in self-efficacy were detected in the other four behaviors between groups. When changes in health behavior were examined between baseline and the 2-year follow-up, it was found that the treatment group exercised more and consumed less dietary fat than the control group. No behavior changes were detected for alcohol consumption, smoking cessation, and weight control. The findings for change in self-efficacy and health behaviors for exercise are consistent and provide partial support for the program's theory of cause and effect (Patrick et al. 1999).

Similar analyses can be performed for moderating variables that might influence program impacts. For example, people who are depressed have lower self-efficacy than people who are not depressed (Grembowski et al. 1993). A longitudinal, explanatory design therefore could be used to determine whether older adults with depression had less changes in self-efficacy and health behavior than older adults without depression.

Did the program's theory of implementation work as expected? As described in Chapter 3, a program may have few impacts because its theory of implementation is faulty. If a program's theory of implementation is defined explicitly in Act I of the evaluation process, the accuracy of the theory can be tested using a longitudinal explanatory design. For example, McGraw et al. (1996) tested the implementation theory of the Child and Adolescent Trial for Cardiovascular Health (CATCH), a multisite, school-based intervention to reduce children's risk for heart disease by changing dietary patterns and physical activity (see Figure 3.3). Their results showed that program implementation was partly inconsistent with the theory, which may provide insights for explaining program impacts.

Are there problems in the organization implementing the program? Because many health programs are implemented by organizations, understanding what goes on inside and between the organizations that run a program is vital to explaining program performance (Chen and Rossi 1983; Grembowski and Blalock 1990). In this approach, a health program is viewed as an *organizational system* composed of interrelated parts that must work together to produce the desired outcomes. To detect the sources and reasons of faulty performance, the organization is broken down into its parts, and each part is examined, as are the relationships among them. Problems often originate in parts that are not working as expected, or where a proper "fit" does not exist among the parts of the organization. Shortell and Kaluzny (2000), Charns and Schaefer (1983), Mintzberg (1983), and Grembowski and Blalock (1990) present organizational models that can be applied to perform a comprehensive assessment of an organization operating a health program.

Explanatory designs are required to perform analyses of organizational systems because several comparisons must be performed to assess the integration, or fit, of the parts of an organization using information from a variety of sources. Cross-sectional analyses can indicate the "health" of the organization at a single point in time; however, programs—and the organizations that implement them—do not "stay in place" but rather change over time (Shortell 1984). Over the life of a 2-year program, personnel enter and leave the organization, protocols change, and sometimes the objectives of the organization or the program itself may change. The advantage of longitudinal designs is their ability to assess how the integration of the organization's parts change over time. For example, when programs are in their infancy, organizational protocols, staff coordination and communication patterns, and information systems may not have jelled and productivity may be low. Later, when the program matures, these start-up problems may no longer exist, and the organization's focus may be improving the quality of the program's services. Tracking and understanding these changes are important because they may be directly related to changes in the program's impacts over time. Grembowski and Blalock (1990) illustrate methods for conducting organizational assessments in program evaluation in more detail.

Questions About Why the Program Had Unintended Consequences

Sometimes programs may have unintended impacts that may or may not be harmful to program participants. Whenever unintended impacts are obtained, detailed evaluations of program implementation may be required to uncover their likely causes. In particular, when a program has harmful consequences, evaluators have an ethical responsibility to identify their reasons to avoid their repetition in the future. Because the aim is to explain unintended results, explanatory designs are essential for this type of evaluation of program implementation.

Unintended consequences occurred in the Medicare demonstration, a preventive program intended to promote and reduce the decline in health in older adults (Patrick et al. 1995; Patrick et al. 1999). Although better health outcomes were expected in the treatment group compared to the control group, the mortality rate at the 2-year follow-up in the treatment group (5.5%) was higher than in the control group (3.3%). At the 4-year follow-up, the gap had closed and was barely significant ($p = .06$). Stratified analyses revealed no significant differences in mortality among adults aged 65 to 74 at either follow-up; however, significant differences in mortality existed among adults aged 75 and over at both follow-ups.

Four alternative explanations of the higher mortality rate in the treatment group were examined:

1. Randomization did not work and treatment group adults were sicker than control group adults.
2. Treatment group adults received a component of the intervention, such as the promotion of exercise or review of medications, which led to higher mortality.
3. A consequence of the autonomy intervention, which was designed to increase living wills and autonomy in decision making at the end of life,

may have successfully promoted self-determination among the treatment group adults.

4. The statistical differences were due to chance; that is, there is no real pattern of higher mortality between the two groups.

The findings revealed that adults in the treatment group were sicker than the adults in control group at baseline for some measures of health status. If multivariable analyses controlled for these differences and the higher mortality rate in the treatment group was no longer significant, then the first explanation would account for the excess mortality. After performing different types of mutivariable analyses, however, the higher mortality remained statistically significant. Turning to the second possible explanation, there were no obvious links between exposure to the preventive services and the excess deaths. In fact, 25% of the treatment group deaths were never exposed to the intervention.

Attention therefore shifted to the third explanation. As a result of the intervention, more living wills were reported in the treatment group (65%) than the control group (47%) at follow-up. Chart reviews of the early treatment group deaths and a sample of control group deaths revealed that a much higher proportion (47%) of the treatment group deaths had Do Not Resuscitate (DNR) orders in their charts. This discovery suggested that by increasing living wills and DNR orders, the intervention may have resulted in higher mortality among the sickest adults in the treatment group.

To test this thinking, the 200 sickest adults from the treatment and control groups were identified from the baseline data. Of these, 36% had a serious medical event, about evenly divided between the treatment and control groups. Of these, adults in the treatment group were more than twice as likely not to receive life-sustaining treatment. Furthermore, complete data from both groups revealed that mortality rates were higher for adults who had a living will (5.6%) than those who did not (3.7%). These findings also are consistent with the previous finding that the excess deaths occurred in the oldest old—adults aged 75 years and older. This evidence supported the conclusion that advance directives contributed to the excess deaths in the treatment group, reflecting the success of the autonomy intervention.

In summary, evaluation of program implementation is an essential element of comprehensive evaluations of health programs. The main purpose is to explain program performance, regardless of whether the program worked, did not work, or had unintended consequences. Such information not only helps decision makers and program administrators manage the program but also contributes to an understanding of what implementation strategies do and do not work and the reasons why.

METHODOLOGICAL ISSUES

A number of methodological issues must be addressed in evaluations of program implementation. Regardless of whether descriptive or explanatory designs are used, or whether quantitative or qualitative methods of data collection are employed, the following methodological questions must be answered:

▶ What is the population of interest?

▶ How will people, organizations, or other units be sampled?

▶ How many cases will be sampled? In what way?

▶ What kinds of comparisons will be made?

▶ What kinds of data will be collected? From whom? When? Using what instruments?

▶ Will the data be available?

▶ What will be done to ensure that the data are reliable and valid?

▶ What kinds of analysis will be conducted? What kinds of findings and statements will result from the analysis?

A common strategy for answering these questions is to use multiple designs and multiple methods of measurement, data collection, and analysis in evaluating the implementation of a program (Shortell 1984). For example, a health clinic serving people from a variety of ethnic and cultural groups may want to know whether its patients are satisfied with their health care. To answer this question, the clinic decides to ask patients to complete a satisfaction questionnaire, translated into different languages, when they visit the clinic. It also conducts focus groups for each of the major cultural groups that visit the clinic to gain more in-depth information about people's opinions about the clinic, and how those opinions might be shaped by cultural beliefs and customs. A third source of information is interviews of interpreters, who were employed by the clinic to improve patient-provider communication and who were well aware of the problems that patients most frequently encountered in the clinic, and why patients from diverse cultures might be dissatisfied about them. If the results of all three methods reveal similar patterns and conclusions, the clinic has greater confidence in the accuracy of the results. This type of inquiry is known as *triangulation* and is a widely used strategy for ensuring the reliability and validity of the findings from evaluations of program implementation.

SUMMARY

If one or more questions are asked about the implementation of a program in Act I of the evaluation process, the next step is to design an evaluation that yields answers for each question. In most cases, the design of an implementation evaluation must be customized to answer the specific questions that are asked about a health program. Implementation evaluations typically use descriptive or explanatory designs that collect cross-sectional and longitudinal data. Most evaluations monitor program implementation either to improve the management of the program or to explain the impacts of the program. To improve rigor, implementation evaluations rely on triangulation, or the use of multiple methods of measurement, data collection, and analysis, to ensure the accuracy of the answer to each question.

Once the designs of an impact or implementation evaluation are chosen, Scene II of the second act begins, where the goal is to develop an evaluation plan and actually conduct the evaluation.

LIST OF TERMS

Descriptive designs

Dose-response effect

Explanatory designs

Health production curve

Implementation designs

Integrity of implementation

Monitoring

Organizational system

Qualitative evaluation

Triangulation

Unintended consequences

STUDY QUESTIONS

1. What types of questions are often asked in evaluations of program implementation?

2. What are the four types of designs for conducting an evaluation of program implementation? Explain why both quantitative and qualitative methods can be used in the four types of designs.

3. What is a program's "hierarchy of objectives," and how can it be used to structure an evaluation of program implementation?

4. Describe three ways of using an evaluation of program implementation to explain the results from an impact evaluation.

5. What methodological issues often confront evaluations of program implementation?

A
C
T
Two

ANSWERING THE QUESTION

Scene 2: ▶ *Planning and Conducting the Evaluation*

Scene 2 marks important accomplishments in the evaluation process. At this point decision makers, administrators, and other interest groups likely have a good understanding of the goals and objectives of the program. They have reached agreement about the purpose of the evaluation and the key questions that it will address. The evaluation designs for answering the questions have been defined and shared with decision makers and other individuals and groups participating in the evaluation process. In short, a well-defined structure for conducting the evaluation now exists, and most people involved agree with it. In many ways, developing this structure is the hardest part of an evaluation and represents a major accomplishment.

Once this milestone is reached, the next work is to plan and conduct the evaluation. That is, given the evaluation questions and the impact and implementation designs for answering them, an evaluation plan containing the details of the designs must be developed. It will serve as a "blueprint" for actually conducting the evaluation in the field. Although there is often a strong temptation to skip developing the evaluation plan and to start immediately collecting and analyzing data, the plan typically is vital to the long-run success of the evaluation. This is because methodological problems exist in almost all evaluations, and the development of a rigorous evaluation plan is the mechanism for identifying and solving these problems before the evaluation begins. Once an evaluation plan is completed and the methodological problems have been worked out, the evaluation is ready to be launched in the field. At this point, the focus shifts to the administration of the evaluation plan, and because most methodological problems have been addressed, the fieldwork is simpler and more straightforward to perform, increasing the likelihood that the evaluation will be accomplished on schedule.

As illustrated in Figure 3.7, the goal of creating an evaluation plan is to establish a tight fit between the design of the evaluation and the detailed methods for executing the design in the field. For almost all evaluations, the methods are divided into the following five sections:

▶ *Populations* the program encompasses and the evaluation will address

▶ *Sampling* cases from those populations through nonrandom sampling or random sampling, if the sizes of the populations are large

▶ *Measurement*, which involves defining the information that will be collected from the populations and samples

▶ *Data collection*, including setting protocols that will obtain the measures for members of the populations and samples

▶ *Data analysis*, including establishing procedures that yield results answering the questions posed in Act I of the evaluation process

These sections apply to both quantitative and qualitative evaluations. For example, if an evaluation asks a question about the impact of the program on health status, how will health status be measured quantitatively? How will the measures of health status be collected? From whom? Similarly, if an evaluation wants to find out why people drop out of a health program by inviting them to focus groups, what will be done to increase their attendance at the focus groups? What qualitative information will be collected in the focus groups?

What will be done with the information after it is collected? In either example, the sections of the evaluation plan must describe in detail how the proposed designs will be carried out.

The five sections are simplest to complete when an evaluation has only a single question and a single design for answering it. Most evaluations, however, have multiple questions that usually require different designs for answering them. In this case, the five sections could be repeated for each design, but this would greatly lengthen the evaluation plan, increase redundancy, and reduce comprehension. A better approach is to develop a plan that has just the five sections, regardless of the number of questions that are asked and the designs for answering them. This approach requires good writing and organizational skills, plus careful thought about how all the pieces of the evaluation fit together. Clearly, the benefits of narrowing the evaluation to a small number of critically important questions in Act I of the evaluation process become evident when writing the evaluation plan!

One way to complete the five sections of the evaluation plan is to perform the following two steps:

Step 1: Outline Each Section. When creating an evaluation plan, the big picture must always be kept in mind. That is, to answer an evaluation question using a given design, how will the evaluation move from point A to point Z? What is the target *population*? Who will be *sampled*? Is the *sample size* large enough to answer each evaluation question? What *information and measures* will be collected about these people? How will the information and measures be *collected*? After the data are collected, how will it be *analyzed*? Outlining each section is a good way to define the basic elements in each section and to verify that the contents of each section fit together in a consistent manner—while also keeping the big picture, or the overall design of the evaluation, in mind. Gordon (1978) presents an outline for planning research projects that is also suitable for many evaluations of health programs.

Step 2: Write Sections in Sequence. With the outline, or big picture, in mind, the second step is to describe in detail the methods that will be performed in each section of the plan. In general, this work is completed more or less in sequence, moving from the population to the data analysis sections of the plan. The opposite order does not work; it is almost impossible to describe the data analysis plan in detail without knowing what the measures are and how they were collected for what people. In moving through the sections, however, it is often necessary to "cycle back" and revise prior sections. For example, developing a mail questionnaire for the data collection section may lead to the discovery that the questionnaire is too long, and therefore the measures section must be revised to reduce the number of items in the questionnaire. In the end, the detailed methods must fit together across the five sections, and these interconnections among the parts are worked out in the course of writing the evaluation plan.

This two-step process is also an excellent strategy for assessing the feasibility of the evaluation's proposed methods. For example, calculating the minimum sample size for an impact evaluation in Step 1 may lead to the discovery that not enough cases exist in the program to perform the impact evaluation that decision makers wanted in Act I of the evaluation process. This news may force decision makers and evaluators to abandon the impact evaluation and focus on questions about the program's implementation.

In Act II of the evaluation process, the evaluator's role and responsibility are to plan and conduct the evaluation. On the one hand, the evaluator becomes a researcher, for the evaluator's work entails the application of evaluation methods to create information that will answer the questions raised in Act I. On the other hand, Act II is not divorced from the interest groups and political issues in Act I, which often permeate into Act II and can influence the evaluator's work. This is particularly true when the evaluator has assumed a participatory, advocacy, or coaching role in Act I of the evaluation process (see Chapter 2). For example, consider the following scenarios, which could arise in the course of conducting an evaluation.

▶ In Act I, the evaluator played a participatory role, working with interest groups to achieve agreement about the evaluation questions. In Act II, the evaluator continues playing this role and holds monthly meetings to report progress and share preliminary results with interest group representatives. In one meeting, early qualitative findings suggest the program might be adversely affecting some program participants. Everyone agrees that the evaluation should be expanded to collect more information about this potential unintended consequence of the program.

▶ An impact evaluation is conducted of a health program using a pretest-posttest control group design. After looking at the pretest results, decision makers inform the evaluator that they do not like the pretest measures anymore, and they want the evaluator to replace them with different ones at the posttest.

▶ An evaluator from outside the agency is hired to perform an impact evaluation of a health program run by the agency. During the course of the evaluation, a group of program staff members privately inform the evaluator that they are "fed up" with the program director, and they want to make sure the evaluator collects process information that will lead to the director's dismissal (Morris 1999).

In short, evaluation is more than the mundane execution of a research plan: It is a "dynamic experience," meaning that evaluation plans may change as new insights are discovered about the program and as this information is shared with decision makers, program staff, and other interest groups. Some changes pose ethical issues, such as a design change that would undermine an impact evaluation or program staff appeals for the evaluator's help that go beyond the impact evaluation that she was hired to do. Application of evaluation's guiding principles can help evaluators solve these and other ethical dilemmas when they occur (Berstene 1999; Davis 1999).

Chapters 7 to 9 provide guidance for developing and implementing the evaluation plan. Chapter 7 presents methods for choosing the program's target populations and describes different sampling techniques for quantitative and qualitative evaluations. Chapter 8 reviews measurement and data collection issues frequently encountered in quantitative and qualitative evaluations. Finally, Chapter 9 describes data analyses for different impact and implementation designs.

CHAPTER 7

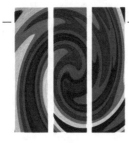

Population and Sampling

Now that the evaluation's questions and the designs for answering them have been defined, the detailed methods for carrying out each design must be developed. This process begins with specifying the *target population*, or the people, organizations, health care systems, or other groups that will contribute information to answer each evaluation question (Fink 1993). In some evaluations, everyone in the target population is included in the evaluation, whereas in other evaluations only members with specific characteristics are included. *Eligibility criteria* define what members of the target population are included or excluded in the evaluation.

Next, depending on the evaluation questions and the methods for answering them, the evaluator must decide whether *random* or *nonrandom sampling* of individuals, organizations, or other groups is necessary. A related issue is whether the expected sample sizes are large enough to answer the evaluation questions. *Quantitative evaluation* of program impacts or implementation typically requires a *minimum* number of eligible members from the target population to draw accurate conclusions. *Qualitative analyses* of program implementation, on the other hand, often can be conducted with a relatively small number of members from a target population. If the size of the eligible target population is too small, the quantitative evaluation may have to be replaced with an evaluation that is more qualitative in nature.

The purpose of this chapter is to describe how to specify the target population(s) of an evaluation, when and how to sample members from a target population, and how to calculate minimum sample size requirements for quantitative evaluations. These procedures are described through the following seven steps:

1. identify the target populations of the evaluation,
2. identify the eligible members of each target population,
3. decide whether random or nonrandom sampling is necessary,
4. choose a nonrandom sample design (if necessary),
5. choose a random sample design (if necessary),
6. calculate sample size requirements, and
7. select the sample.

STEP 1: IDENTIFY THE TARGET POPULATIONS OF THE EVALUATION

The target populations of an evaluation typically are found in the questions posed about the program in Act I of the evaluation process. The first task, therefore, is to identify the population in each of the questions.

For example, suppose that a 4-year high school with 1,200 students, or 300 students in each grade, has implemented a teen clinic staffed by a nurse practitioner and a mental health specialist at the start of the school year. At the end of the school year, an evaluation is conducted to answer the following questions:

A. What percentage of students saw the clinic nurse or the mental health specialist at least once during the school year?
B. Are the utilization percentages similar or different across the four grades?
C. What student characteristics are associated with use of the teen clinic?

In this evaluation, the target population consists of all teenagers from all grades who were enrolled at the high school at any time in the current school year. Let's assume, however, that the school district and the high school have a formal policy that students can participate in research projects only if their parents and guardians permit them to do so. Parents and guardians are an *adjunct population* that must provide consent before the members of the target population—that is, the high school students themselves—can participate in the evaluation.

For a second example, the following impact and implementation questions might be asked about the Medicare demonstration at Group Health Cooperative of Puget Sound, which provided a package of preventive services to older adults (Grembowski et al. 1993; Patrick et al. 1999; the demonstration is described in greater detail in Chapter 3):

D. What is the effect of the package of preventive services on the health behaviors of Medicare enrollees at Group Health Cooperative of Puget Sound?

E. Are the physicians and nurses who delivered the package of preventive services to Medicare enrollees in the treatment group satisfied with the program?

Each question targets a different population. In question D, the target population consists of Medicare enrollees who are members of Group Health Cooperative of Puget Sound for at least 1 year before the start date of the demonstration. In question E, the population is composed of the physicians and nurses at Group Health Cooperative who delivered the package of services to the Medicare enrollees in the intervention group.

STEP 2: IDENTIFY THE ELIGIBLE MEMBERS OF EACH TARGET POPULATION

Once the target populations are identified, the next step is to identify the individuals in each population who will be asked to participate in the evaluation. In some evaluations, all members of the target population are included in the actual evaluation (Fink 1993). In the evaluation of the high school clinic described earlier, the evaluation might include all teenagers enrolled at the high school as its target population. Similarly, an evaluation of a prenatal care class for pregnant teenagers might decide to include everyone who registered for the class, regardless of actual attendance.

In other evaluations, only members of the target population with specific characteristics are included in the evaluation, and by definition, members who do not have these characteristics are excluded from the evaluation. The criteria for *inclusion* and *exclusion*, or *eligibility*, are "filters" that define who is and who is not a member of an evaluation's target population. Members of a target population may be included or excluded from an evaluation based on several criteria, such as their

▶ Personal characteristics, such as age, gender, and marital status

▶ Professional characteristics, such as being a physician, nurse, or dentist

▶ Geographic factors, such as where a person lives or was born

▶ Literacy (the ability to read and write in a given language)

▶ Presence or absence of a telephone where a person can be contacted

▶ Presence or absence of health insurance, or the type of health insurance

▶ Health behaviors, such as smoking or amount of exercise

▶ Health status

▶ Presence or absence of one or more medical conditions

The inclusion and exclusion criteria imposed on a target population are important because they essentially determine the generalizability of the future findings of the evaluation. If members of the target population with specific characteristics are excluded from the evaluation, the findings of the evaluation cannot be generalized to other people with those characteristics.

Returning to the school clinic example, although we may want to include all students from all grades who were enrolled at the high school at any time in the current school year, some students inevitably will be excluded from the evaluation. First and foremost, if a parent or guardian does not consent to a student participating in the evaluation, the student must be excluded from the evaluation. Second, if students leave the high school before the end of the school year, the evaluator may decide to exclude those students from the evaluation. Third, if data will be collected through a self-administered questionnaire written in English, students who cannot read and write in English are excluded as well. Fourth, if students are asked to complete the questionnaires while at school, students who are absent are excluded from the evaluation.

These four inclusion-exclusion criteria provide some examples of why all members of the target population may not be included in the evaluation. Given that only a subset of the target population is included in the evaluation, an immediate concern is whether excluding members of the target population will influence the findings of the evaluation. For example, let's suppose that students who are absent due to illness are excluded from the evaluation, and these students also have never visited the high school clinic. The clinic utilization rates calculated from students who completed the questionnaire in class will there-fore likely be "too high"—that is, the percentage of students using the clinic would be lower if these absent students also had completed a questionnaire. In short, the consequences of including and excluding certain members of the tar-get population from the evaluation merit careful review before the data collec-tion process is carried out.

Inclusion and exclusion criteria also exist for the Medicare demonstration. In question D, the population is defined as all Medicare enrollees at Group Health Cooperative of Puget Sound when the demonstration began, which in 1988 was about 40,000 older adults. All the Medicare enrollees did not partici-pate in the program, however. Only a minority of the Medicare enrollees partic-ipated in the demonstration, based on specific inclusion and exclusion criteria, which are illustrated in the participant recruitment tree in Figure 7.1.

The Medicare enrollee population is indicated at the top of the tree. Several branches appear on the trunk of the tree, and each branch defines a specific cri-terion that either includes or excludes enrollees from the demonstration. The first branch near the top of the tree addresses the first inclusion-exclusion crite-rion, the medical center where enrollees receive their health care. Group Health operates several medical centers in the Seattle metropolitan area, and Medicare enrollees are distributed unevenly across the centers. Because it was not feasible to launch the demonstration in all centers, four medical centers with large num-bers of Medicare enrollees were chosen as demonstration sites. In addition, be-cause the evaluation required information about each person's utilization of health services in the year prior to the demonstration, Medicare enrollees must be members of the cooperative for at least 1 year. Therefore, 31,375 Medicare enrollees who did *not* receive their health care from the four centers and had less than 1 year of enrollment at Group Health Cooperative were *excluded* from the demonstration (shown *below* the trunk of the tree), and 8,703 en-rollees who received their health care from the four centers were *included* in the demonstration (shown above the trunk of the tree).

Moving down to the next branch on the tree, of the remaining 8,703 en-rollees, 2,159 enrollees who had few physician visits were excluded from the demonstration, while 6,544 enrollees with higher physician visits were included in the demonstration. This criterion was imposed because older adults with few physician visits were probably healthier than adults with more physician visits, and the preventive service package would likely have greater health benefits for older adults with more physician visits.

Although the majority of primary care physicians at the four centers partici-pated in the demonstration, some physicians declined to do so. The third branch indicates that 824 enrollees of nonparticipating physicians were ex-

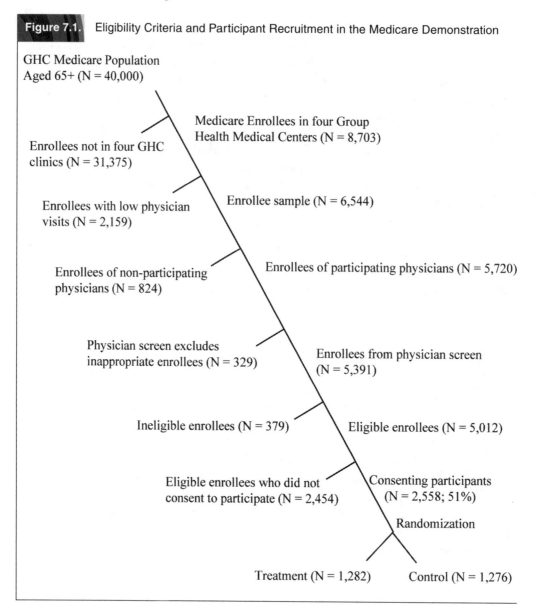

Figure 7.1.   Eligibility Criteria and Participant Recruitment in the Medicare Demonstration

GHC Medicare Population
Aged 65+ (N = 40,000)

Medicare Enrollees in four Group
Health Medical Centers (N = 8,703)

Enrollees not in four GHC
clinics (N = 31,375)

Enrollees with low physician
visits (N = 2,159)

Enrollee sample (N = 6,544)

Enrollees of non-participating
physicians (N = 824)

Enrollees of participating physicians (N = 5,720)

Physician screen excludes
inappropriate enrollees (N = 329)

Enrollees from physician screen
(N = 5,391)

Ineligible enrollees (N = 379)

Eligible enrollees (N = 5,012)

Eligible enrollees who did not
consent to participate (N = 2,454)

Consenting participants
(N = 2,558; 51%)

Randomization

Treatment (N = 1,282)   Control (N = 1,276)

cluded from the demonstration, and that 5,720 Medicare enrollees of the participating physicians were included in the study.

Because of extremely poor health, some of the 5,720 Medicare enrollees might not be suitable candidates for the package of preventive services. Participating physicians reviewed their Medicare patients and excluded 329 enrollees whose health status would likely prohibit their participation, leaving 5,391 enrollees. Finally, 379 enrollees were found to be ineligible for the program for various reasons, leaving 5,012 Medicare enrollees who were invited to participate in the demonstration. About half consented to do so ($N = 2,558$), and they were randomized into the treatment and control groups.

Clearly, the 5,012 Medicare enrollees who were invited to participate in the demonstration were not randomly sampled from the target population, and therefore the findings of the evaluation cannot be generalized to the target population of 40,000 Medicare enrollees at Group Health Cooperative in 1988, nor can they be generalized to other Medicare enrollees in the Seattle metropolitan area or in other areas of the United States. For similar reasons, the evaluation's findings based on 2,558 consenting adults cannot be generalized to the subgroup of 5,012 Medicare enrollees who were invited to participate in the demonstration. Patrick et al. (1999) and Durham et al. (1991) compared the characteristics of participants and nonparticipants and found that nonparticipants tended to be older, live farther from their clinics, and have fewer physician visits. Findings generally showed that invited enrollees with the very best and very worst health status were less likely to participate in the demonstration. In short, the findings of the demonstration can be generalized only to those older adults who were invited and consented to participate in the demonstration.

In the evaluation of the high school clinic and the Medicare demonstration, a roster exists indicating all members of the evaluation's target population. In some evaluations, however, the program or agency may not have records indicating the people who received program services. This is often the case for health programs serving "hidden" or "hard-to-reach" populations. For example, in most needle exchange programs for drug addicts, syringes are exchanged anonymously, and thus the program typically does not have records of who received its services or a list of drug addicts in the community. Similarly, community programs for homeless people or HIV-infected individuals may not have a list of all homeless or infected people in the community.

In this context, alternative methods must be employed for identifying eligible members of the target population. For example, Burt (1996) describes alternative methods for identifying the homeless in a community, such as identifying individuals in homeless shelters or living in public places, which may be used independently or in combination with each other. Alternatively, the evaluation may identify eligible members in ways that do not rely on a census of a target population in a community. For example, in a needle exchange program, the evaluation's eligible target population might be defined as all individuals who exchange syringes on randomly selected days in a specific month of the year. A key assumption of this approach is that individuals who exchange syringes on these days are similar to individuals who exchange syringes on other days of the year, which may or may not be the case.

STEP 3: DECIDE WHETHER RANDOM OR NONRANDOM SAMPLING IS NECESSARY

The next step is to decide whether to sample members from each target population. If the target population of the evaluation is relatively small, sampling may not be warranted. For example, a prenatal care class for pregnant teenagers may have a small number of people enrolled in the class. Because the evaluation's target population is small, an implementation evaluation can include all class members, and sampling is unnecessary.

If the target population of the evaluation is large, *random sampling* may be warranted (Aday 1996; Salant and Dillman 1994). In random sampling, which is a type of probability sampling, each member of the target population has a known probability of being sampled. Because the probability of being sampled is known, the sample estimate of a characteristic in the target population can be calculated with a known level of accuracy, which is defined by the amount of sampling error. This is an important attribute if the goal is to estimate a characteristic of a larger population.

The main reason for random sampling is efficiency (Salant and Dillman 1994). Sampling members of the population reduces the cost of data collection while also estimating the value of a characteristic in the population. Because of this feature, random sampling is often vital for evaluations that have a limited budget for data collection. As a final point, note that "random sampling" from a target population is a different concept from the "random assignment" of individuals to the intervention and control groups in an experimental impact evaluation (see Chapter 4).

In contrast, in *nonrandom sampling*, which also is known as nonprobability or purposive sampling, members of the target population are selected for subjective reasons, such as that the members are convenient to interview, the members had the best outcome in the intervention group, or the members are thought to be "typical" of people in the program. The advantage of nonrandom sampling is the ability to collect data from individuals who are most relevant to answering an evaluation question. Its major disadvantage is that each member of the target population has an unknown probability of being included in the sample. For this reason, a nonrandom sample cannot be used to estimate the value of a characteristic in the target population with a known level of accuracy.

Different methods exist for performing nonrandom and random sampling. These are reviewed in the next sections.

STEP 4: CHOOSE A NONRANDOM SAMPLE DESIGN (IF NECESSARY)

If nonrandom sampling of members from the target population is necessary to answer one or more evaluation questions, the next step is to choose a nonrandom sampling design that is most appropriate for answering each question. For example, in the evaluation of the high school clinic, the evaluators may decide to conduct focus groups to answer the following evaluation question: "For students with no clinic visits, what reasons do students give for not visiting the clinic?" To sample students for the focus groups, the evaluators consider the following list of nonrandom sampling designs (Miles and Huberman 1984; Patton 1987; Simon 1969).

Quota sampling: In this method of sampling, people who are "typical" of a subgroup are selected until a predetermined "quota" is reached. For example, a city may be divided into quarters, and an interviewer is sent to each quarter to interview "typical" female homeless adults, until a quota of 10 interviews are collected in each quarter.

Extreme or deviant case sampling: Cases that are at the opposite ends of a continuum are sampled to gain insights about program performance. Examples include treatment group members who completed the program vs. those who dropped out of the program, program staff with high vs. low morale, or program sites with busy vs. idle waiting rooms.

Maximum variation sampling: This technique selects cases that vary as much as possible. The heterogenous sample is used in qualitative evaluations that seek to find underlying themes or patterns that are common to a wide variety of program participants.

Homogeneous sampling: This type of sampling often is performed using focus groups and other qualitative methods where the goal is to collect in-depth information from people with similar characteristics.

Typical case sampling: If the goal of the evaluation is to describe the typical experiences of people in the program, a small number of more or less "typical" program participants may be sampled from program records or the recommendations of program staff. This type of sampling is performed, for example, to describe the "typical case" to those who are unfamiliar with the program, recognizing that findings cannot be generalized to all program participants.

Critical case sampling: The aim of this technique is to sample cases that are strategically important for understanding program performance. For example, if a program is implemented in many sites, the site with the best track record might be sampled as a critical case, with the assumption that if the program does not work in this ideal setting, it may not work elsewhere.

Snowball, chain, or network sampling: This technique begins by asking key informants to identify people who are knowledgeable about some aspect of the program, then asking those people the same question. After repeating this cycle several times, the list converges on a small number of people that most people mention, and the list becomes the sample for the evaluation.

Criterion sampling: Cases are selected that meet a specific criterion for in-depth study. For example, in a program to reduce hypertension, adults who do not improve are selected for in-depth analysis.

Confirmatory and disconfirming case sampling: When the preliminary findings of an evaluation are known, "confirming" cases may be selected to illustrate the patterns. Alternatively, "disconfirming" cases may be selected as rival interpretations, to qualify the findings, or to cross-check the accuracy of the preliminary findings.

Convenience sampling: In this technique, cases are sampled in a fast and convenient way. Because this form of sampling has no underlying purpose, its cases may not provide critical information for the evaluation, and therefore this form of sampling is not recommended.

Next, the evaluators consider the requirements of conducting successful focus groups. In general, focus groups should have a degree of homogeneity but also some variation to ensure differences in opinion (Krueger 1994), which may (in a study of students) encompass such factors as whether the students

▶ Are from the same grade or different grades

▶ Have the same personal characteristics (such as whether the groups should be composed of only males, only females, or both)

▶ Speak the same language

▶ Saw only the clinic nurse, only the mental health specialist, or both

On the basis of these considerations, the list of nonrandom sampling designs, and their evaluation question, the evaluators decide to employ a combination of quota/homogeneous sampling. Students without clinic visits are the basis of homogenous sampling. Then, eight focus groups are planned, two groups for each of the four grades in the high school, with separate focus groups for males and females in each grade. Quota sampling will be employed to identify 10 "typical" students for each group (Krueger 1994).

Depending on the evaluation questions asked about a program, some evaluations gather qualitative information from multiple target populations using one or more sampling methods, then use triangulation to identify patterns and trends across the populations. For example, the Medicare demonstration could conduct separate focus groups to find out what older adults in the treatment group thought about the package of preventive services, to find out what the physicians and nurses who delivered the preventive services thought about the program, and to find out what clinic and program staff who ran the program thought about it. This qualitative assessment entails three target populations— Medicare enrollees and providers in the treatment group, as well as program staff—and different nonrandom sampling designs might be used to select members for each focus group.

STEP 5: CHOOSE A RANDOM SAMPLE DESIGN (IF NECESSARY)

If random sampling of members from the target population appears necessary, the next step is to choose a random sampling design that is most appropriate for answering an evaluation question. Alternative random sampling designs vary considerably in their complexity, feasibility, and implications for data analysis. The following five sampling designs, which occur relatively often in health program evaluation, are reviewed in this section: simple and systematic random sampling, proportionate stratified sampling, disproportionate stratified sampling, post-stratification sampling, and cluster sampling (Aday 1996; Blalock 1972; Kish 1965; Snedecor and Cochran 1980).

Simple and Systematic Random Sampling

In simple random sampling, perhaps the most widely used sampling design in program evaluation, each member of the target population as well as all combinations of members have an equal probability of being selected. One way of performing a simple random sample is to create a list of all members in the target population and randomly select members from the list by lottery (picking members out of a hat) or using a random numbers table or computer-generated list of random numbers until the minimum sample size is attained. Aday (1996), Salant and Dillman (1994), and other survey and sampling texts provide guidelines for drawing a sample from a random numbers table.

This sample design is relatively simple to perform and assumes that a list of all members of the target population is available. If a list of the population members is not available, a simple random sample cannot be performed, and an alternative sampling design must be chosen, such as cluster sampling, which is described later. An exception to this rule might occur, for example, in the evaluation of a mass media campaign to reduce smoking, where the evaluation wants to find out what percentage of adults in the community have heard or seen the campaign's postings in newspapers, on the radio, and so forth. In this case, a survey that sampled working telephone numbers through random digit dialing—a type of simple random sampling—could be performed (Salant and Dillman 1994). Because only people with telephones have a probability of being interviewed, the survey findings would not be generalizable to people without telephones.

Systematic random sampling, an alternative method of choosing an equal probability sample, is a substitute for simple random sampling and is often easier to perform in the field. Systematic random sampling also requires a list of all members of the target population and a minimum sample size. For example, suppose that you want to sample 400 students from a high school containing 1,200 students. In a systematic random sample, a sampling interval is calculated by dividing the population size by the sample size, which produces a sampling interval of 3 (3 = 1,200/400) in this example. A random numbers table is used to pick a number at random between the values of 1 and 3. For the first three students in the list of all students, this random number identifies the student who is sampled first (for example, if the number "2" is chosen randomly, the second student in the list is selected). Given this random start point, every third student is sampled systematically through the end of the list, yielding a sample size of 400 students.

Although both simple random sampling and systematic sampling yield unbiased estimates of population means, their sample variances are slightly biased estimates of the population variance, when random sampling is performed without replacement or the sample size is small. Data collected with simple or systematic random samples can be analyzed readily by most statistical software.

Proportionate Stratified Sampling

Compared to other sampling designs, simple random sample and systematic sample estimates of population parameters may not be the most "efficient." The efficiency of a sample estimate, such as the sample mean, refers to how much the sampling distribution is clustered about the true mean of the target population. The degree of clustering is measured by the standard error: The smaller the standard error, the greater the efficiency of the sample estimate. Stratified sampling is one method of increasing the efficiency of sample estimates. In stratified sampling, the population is first divided into mutually exclusive, homogeneous groups according to some criterion, and then independent samples are drawn from each group. To the degree that strata are more homogeneous than the population from which they are chosen, between-strata variation is eliminated, leaving only within-strata variation as a source of sampling error. Because all simple random samples contain both sources of sampling error, stratified sampling is normally more efficient than a simple random sampling design.

Stratified sampling, however, produces more efficient estimates only if the strata are homogeneous. If the strata are as heterogeneous as might be expected in a simple random sample, stratified sampling is not more efficient than simple random sampling. In other words, if the differences between the strata (e.g., as measured by strata means) are small compared to the within-strata differences, nothing is gained through stratification. If, however, the criterion for stratifying the population (for example, high school class) is highly related to the variable studied (for example, whether a student saw a health professional in the high school clinic), stratified sampling may be considerably more efficient than simple random sampling.

In proportional stratified sampling, constant sampling fractions are used across strata, producing sample strata directly proportional to the stratum's population size. For example, if the freshman, sophomore, junior, and senior classes form four separate strata, respectively containing 400, 350, 300, and 250 students, a proportional stratified sample using a 1/5 sampling fraction across all four strata would yield proportional sample strata of sizes 80, 70, 60, and 50, respectively. By controlling the number of cases that fall into each stratum, proportional stratified sampling ensures a more representative sample than might be expected using a simple random sample—a benefit yielding greater accuracy in later data analysis. If the size of a simple random sample is large, however, chance alone usually ensures approximately the correct proportions from each of the strata, making stratified sampling unnecessary.

In general, proportional stratified sampling has a number of desirable features. First, it often yields modest gains in reduced variances. If proportional stratified sampling is used with cluster sampling, the gains may be even greater. Second, it's safe: The variances of a proportional stratified sample cannot be greater than variances in an unstratified sample of the same size. Third, it is usually easy to do. Fourth, formulas for estimating population means are self-weighting; complex statistical formulas are unnecessary.

Disproportionate Stratified Sampling

Although disproportionate stratified sampling is neither safe, self-weighting, nor simple to do, it improves efficiency over both the proportional stratified sampling and simple random sampling designs. In disproportionate stratified sampling, different sampling fractions are used across population strata to manipulate the number of cases selected in each stratum. This sampling design is often used when the evaluator wants to compare one stratum with another. For example, the racial/ethnic mix of students in a high school may be unbalanced, such as 300 students having a Hispanic background and 700 students being white, and the evaluation wants to compare utilization of the high school clinic between the two groups. If the comparison requires a sample of 200 students in each racial group, a sampling fraction of approximately 2/7 for the white students and 2/3 for the Hispanic students would produce equal-sized strata, allowing accurate comparisons between strata.

Disproportionate stratified sampling should be used only when the standard deviations within separate strata differ greatly (that is, when differences are several-fold), or when data-gathering costs differ greatly between strata, or when the principal variable is highly skewed or has an asymmetrical distribution. In these cases, maximum efficiency is achieved by making the sampling fraction for each stratum directly proportional to the standard deviation within the stratum and inversely proportional to the square root of the cost of data collection for each case within the stratum.

As in proportional stratified sampling, this design also requires homogeneous strata. Although a stratum may be homogeneous for one variable, however, other variables in the stratum will most likely be more heterogeneous. In evaluations involving more than one variable, it may be difficult to identify a set of sampling fractions that will yield the smallest sampling error for a given cost for all variables in the study. In these situations, a design that maximizes efficiency for one variable may be extremely inefficient for another, and the safe approach may be a proportional stratified sampling design.

After drawing a disproportionate sample, the evaluation also may want to generalize its findings back to the target population. Because sampling fractions vary across strata, the sample data must be "weighted" using the disproportionate sampling fractions to create a composite picture of the population. Procedures for weighting samples are described in Aday (1996), Salant and Dillman (1994), and other survey and sampling textbooks.

Post-Stratification Sampling

Cases selected through a simple random sample may be categorized into strata at a later date. Estimates of population means and variances are calculated from the newly stratified sampled cases through weighting procedures, as described in Kish (1965). In this post-stratification sampling design, information on the proportion of the population in each stratum and the criteria for classifying the sample cases into the strata must be available. The criteria for classifying cases must be the same in both the sample and the population to avoid bias.

A second type of post-stratification design also exists. Stratified sampling normally involves sorting the population into strata and then sampling from these strata lists. If this sorting procedure is too expensive, but the proportion of the population in each stratum as well as selection criteria are known and accessible, cases may be drawn from the population through simple random sampling and categorized into the appropriate strata until each sample stratum has been filled with the desired number of cases. This approach may be used in either the proportional or the disproportional stratification designs.

Cluster Sampling

In most of the previous sampling designs, a list of members in the target population must be available. In some health programs, an accurate list of population members may not exist, or if a list does exist, it may be out of date or contain inaccurate information. In addition, if the evaluation requires personal interviews of members of the target population, there may be insufficient resources to conduct the interviews through the previous sampling designs. Cluster sampling is one approach for solving these problems.

Cluster sampling divides a target population into a large number of groups, or clusters, which are sampled randomly using one or more of the previous sampling designs. In single-stage cluster sampling, clusters may be selected through a simple random sample, and then every member of the cluster is selected for the evaluation. In multistage sampling, where sampling is performed more than once, a simple random sample of clusters may be performed, and then a simple random sample of the members in each cluster also may be conducted until minimum sample size requirements are satisfied. For example, suppose an evaluator wants to conduct personal interviews about a mass media campaign to reduce smoking in a large city. First-stage cluster sampling can be performed, for example, by identifying all the city's census tracts with residences, then randomly selecting census tracts for the sample. Multistage cluster sampling is performed, for example, by randomly sampling blocks in each sampled cluster, and then randomly sampling every third dwelling unit in the sampled blocks, and then randomly sampling every second adult in each of those dwelling units to be interviewed.

In most cases, cluster samples are less efficient (that is, they have greater variances and sampling errors) than simple random samples of the same size, but the cluster sample will cost much less than the simple random sample to perform. The efficiency of a cluster design depends on cluster size and how homogeneous the members of the cluster are. Intraclass correlation is a measure of homogeneity among the members of the cluster. As the homogeneity of the cluster increases, so does the amount of intraclass correlation, and the cluster design becomes less efficient. If a cluster is homogeneous, a small (cluster) sample size can be selected to estimate the cluster mean. If the cluster is heterogeneous, there is less intraclass correlation, and larger samples of cluster members are required. In most cases, the aim of cluster sampling is to select clusters that are as heterogeneous as possible because doing so reduces intraclass correlation, which increases the efficiency of the cluster design. Because larger clusters tend to be more heterogeneous and therefore have less intraclass correlation than smaller clusters, sampling from larger clusters is one way to increase heterogeneity.

If random sampling is necessary, the evaluator picks one of the above random sampling designs that is most appropriate for answering the evaluation questions of a specific program. The simple sampling designs described above can be performed readily in most health program evaluations. As the complexity of the design increases, so does the need for advice from a statistician with expertise in sample design.

Regardless of the random sampling design that is chosen, the evaluator must decide how large a sample to draw. This issue is addressed in the next section.

STEP 6: CALCULATE SAMPLE SIZE REQUIREMENTS

In general, a health program may use quantitative or qualitative methods (or both) to answer one or more evaluation questions. In quantitative evaluations, a key issue is the *sample size*, or the number of individuals (or organizations, communities, or other groups) that are included in data collection and analysis (as described later in Chapters 8 and 9). When quantitative data are collected for all eligible members of a target population or through random or nonrandom sampling, the data usually must be collected from a minimum number of individuals to satisfy the statistical requirements of the data analysis. Thus, before the sample can be drawn and the data can be collected, the *minimum sample size requirements* for the data analysis must be determined.

Methods for calculating minimum sample sizes are reviewed in this section. These methods generally do not apply to qualitative methods of data collection and analysis, which typically can be conducted with small sample sizes. An exception to this rule occurs when *representative* qualitative data collection is an important aspect of the evaluation. For example, high schools may implement a new curriculum to promote healthy behavior among students (McGraw et al. 1996), and in-class observation of the new curriculum is an essential element of the program's implementation evaluation. In this design, the classrooms are the target population, and the goal is to obtain representative findings by randomly sampling class sessions for observation using one of the random sampling designs described earlier. If quantitative measures of classroom teaching are derived from the qualitative observations, the minimum number of classroom sessions must be calculated using methods described in this section.

Types of Sample Size Calculations

Calculating minimum sample size requirements begins with the questions that an evaluation is supposed to answer. In general, two basic types of evaluation questions exist. The first type consists of *descriptive* questions about what is going on within the program. These are asked commonly in evaluations of program implementation. For example, question A (see p. 170) asks what percentage of students saw the clinic nurse or the mental health specialist at least once during the school year.

The second type consists of *comparative* questions, which, as the name implies, compare the characteristics of one group with the characteristics of another group to find out if the two groups are similar or different. Comparative questions are common in evaluations of program implementation. For example, question B (p. 170) compares clinic utilization to see if the percentages of students who visited the clinic at least once are similar or different across the four grades. In the Medicare demonstration, a comparative question might ask whether Medicare enrollees who are female are more satisfied with the preventive services than enrollees who are male. By definition, impact evaluations ask comparative questions, such as question D (p. 171), which compares the health status of the Medicare enrollees in the treatment group with the health status of enrollees in the control group.

Descriptive and comparative questions have different methods for calculating sample sizes, which are described in the sections that follow. When an evaluation asks only one descriptive question or one comparative question, the calculation of the sample size is straightforward. When an evaluation asks several descriptive and comparative questions, each question may require a different sample size to answer it. In this case, which sample size should be chosen? One strategy for handling this dilemma is to pick the most important question of the evaluation and calculate the sample size for answering that question. The disadvantage with this strategy is that sample sizes may be too small to answer the other questions, which may be a problem if decision makers truly demand answers for them. An alternative strategy is to calculate the sample size for each question and use the largest one, which ensures that an adequate number of cases exists to answer all the questions of the evaluation. When an evaluation's budget is too small to collect data for the largest sample size, some combination of these two strategies may be used to achieve an acceptable sample size for the evaluation.

Sample Size Calculations for Descriptive Questions

The sample size for answering a descriptive question depends on the following three factors:

▶ The *precision* or accuracy of the answer, which depends on the amount of sampling error

▶ The *population size*

▶ The *variation* of the characteristic in the population

Table 7.1 presents *minimum* sample sizes to estimate population percentages, depending on the amount of sampling error, the population size, and the variation of the characteristic (Salant and Dillman 1994). For example, let's suppose you wanted to answer question A about the teen clinics in the high school: What percentage of students saw the clinic nurse or the mental health specialist at least once during the school year? Let's assume that after the inclusion and exclusion criteria are applied, 1,000 students are asked to complete a questionnaire about the teen clinic. Let's also assume that utilization of the clinic has little variation; some teenagers—about 20%—used the clinic, and most teenagers—about 80%—did not use the clinic. Given a population of 1,000 teenagers and a 20-80 split on clinic utilization, the 5th row of Table 7.1 indicates that a minimum sample size of 406 teenagers is required to estimate the percentage of teenagers who utilized the clinic in the population within a range of ±3%, at the 95% confidence level. That is, 19 out of 20 times we can expect that the percentage of teenagers who visited the clinic in the population will fall within the range of the sample's estimate ±3%. Therefore, if you conducted the survey and found that 23% of teenagers had visited a nurse or mental health specialist in the clinic, the chances are that 19 out of 20 times the population's actual utilization is within ±3% of this estimate, or between 20% and 26%.

Suppose, however, that the teenagers were enthusiastic about the clinic and that clinic utilization varied more than expected, with 50% of the teens using the clinic and 50% not using the clinic. With greater variation, the 50-50 split would require a minimum sample size of 516 students to estimate clinic utilization in the target population, within a range of ±3% at a 95% confidence level.

Alternatively, suppose that you only wanted to know *roughly* what percentage of students were using the clinic, and therefore you could tolerate a less precise estimate of this characteristic. You therefore increase the amount of sampling error from 3% to 5%. Assuming a 20-80 split in clinic utilization in the population, a minimum sample size of 198 teenagers is required to estimate clinic utilization in the population with a range of ±5%. Again, if even less accuracy is required, the sampling error might be increased to 10%, and assuming a 20-80 split, a minimum sample size of 58 teenagers is necessary to estimate the population value within ±10%.

TABLE 7.1 Minimum Sample Sizes Needed for Various Population Sizes and Characteristics, at Three Levels of Precision (95% confidence level)

Population Size	±3% Sampling Error		±5% Sampling Error		±10% Sampling Error	
	50/50 Split	80/20 Split	50/50 Split	80/20 Split	50/50 Split	80/20 Split
100	92	87	80	71	49	38
250	203	183	152	124	70	49
500	341	289	217	165	81	55
750	441	358	254	185	85	57
1,000	516	406	278	198	88	58
2,500	748	537	333	224	93	60
5,000	880	601	357	234	94	61
10,000	964	639	370	240	95	61
25,000	1,023	665	378	234	96	61
50,000	1,045	674	381	245	96	61
100,000	1,056	678	383	245	96	61
1,000,000	1,066	682	384	246	96	61
100,000,000	1,067	683	384	246	96	61

SOURCE: Salant P, Dillman DA. *How to Conduct Your Own Survey.* © Copyright 1997 by John Wiley & Sons, Inc. Reprinted with permission of John Wiley & Sons, Inc.

In all these examples, the sample sizes refer to the number of completed and returned questionnaires. The sample size therefore must be increased to account for people who do not return their completed questionnaires. For example, if the minimum sample size is 406 students and we expect that 80% of the students will complete the questionnaire, the sample size must be increased to 508 (406/.80 = 508 after rounding) to obtain 406 completed questionnaires.

In addition, population size has two important implications for calculating minimum sample sizes (Salant and Dillman 1994). First, minimum sample sizes are similar for large populations. Once the population exceeds 25,000, sample sizes vary little, regardless of whether the population is composed of 100,000 or 100,000,000 people. If Congress changed the Medicare program and wanted to find out what Medicare enrollees across the nation thought about the changes, a sample size of 1,100 to 1,200 interviews would be sufficient, assuming a conservative 50-50 split in opinions about the changes.

The second implication is that sampling may not be warranted in small populations. If a program's target population has 250 or less people, over 80% of them must be sampled, assuming a 50-50 split and ±3% sampling error. In this case, sampling will not greatly reduce the cost of data collection, and data collection from all members of the target population may be a better course. When working with small program populations, the averages and variances reflect population parameters, and the sample size calculations for descriptive questions do not apply.

Sample Size Calculations for Comparative Questions

Question B about the teen clinic asks whether the percentages of students who visited the clinic in the school year are similar or different across the four grades. If a difference in percentages exists, the difference likely will be the greatest between the freshmen (9th graders) and seniors (12th graders) for various reasons, such as maturity, years of high school attendance, and other factors, and we expect freshmen to have lower utilization than seniors.

To find out whether the clinic utilization percentages are similar or different, we draw a sample and collect sample data measuring the clinic utilization percentages for freshmen and seniors. In the data analysis, a *null hypothesis* is posed stating that no difference exists between the clinic utilization percentages of freshmen and seniors. Based on sample data, a statistical test of the null hypothesis is performed, and if the test is statistically significant, we *reject* the null hypothesis and conclude that the clinic utilization rates are different from each other, and that the difference is not due to chance. If the statistical test is not statistically significant, we do *not* reject the null hypothesis, and we conclude that the clinic utilization rates are not different from each other.

How can we tell if the results of the statistical test are accurate? One way is to compare the conclusion of the statistical test based on sample data with the true utilization percentages in the population (Lipsey 1990, 1998). Four possibilities exist: There *is* or *is not* a true difference in the utilization percentages of the freshmen and senior populations, and the statistical test on the sample data either *is* or *is not* significant. The combinations of the four possibilities are presented in Table 7.2. The upper-left cell contains a correct conclusion: A true difference exists between the freshmen and senior populations, and a significant difference is detected in the statistical test. The lower-right cell also contains a

TABLE 7.2   The Possibilities of Error in Statistical Significance Tests for Differences Between Two Groups

Conclusion From Statistical Test on Sample Data	Population Circumstances	
	Group A and Group B Differ	Group A and Group B Do Not Differ
Significant difference (reject null hypothesis)	*Power* Correct conclusion Probability = $1 - \beta$	Type I error Probability = α
No significant difference (fail to reject null hypothesis)	Type II error Probability = β	Correct conclusion Probability = $1 - \alpha$

SOURCE: Lipsey MW. *Design Sensitivity: Statistical Power for Experimental Research.* © Copyright 1990 by Sage Publications, Inc. Reprinted by permission of Sage Publications, Inc.

correct conclusion: No difference exists in the population, and no significant difference is detected in the statistical test.

In contrast, incorrect conclusions are drawn in the lower-left and upper-right cells. These indicate the two types of error that are possible in statistical significance tests. The upper-right cell contains a Type I error, or the risk of finding a statistically significant difference in the clinic utilization percentages for freshmen and seniors when, in fact, the two groups do not differ. This risk, or probability, is symbolized by the Greek letter α. By convention, researchers set α to .05, which indicates the maximum acceptable probability of a Type I error (Lipsey 1998). Thus, if the null hypothesis is true, the probability of incorrectly rejecting the null hypothesis is 5%, or 1 out of 20 times.

The lower-left cell contains a Type II error, or the risk of finding no significant difference between the clinic utilization percentages for freshmen and seniors when, in fact, they actually are different. This risk, or probability, is indicated by the Greek letter β. Thus, if the null hypothesis is false, the probability of failing to reject the null hypothesis is defined by β. *Statistical power* is the probability $(1 - \beta)$ that a significant difference will be detected *if* one actually exists between the populations (as shown in the upper-left cell).

Our goal is to *maximize* statistical power. That is, if a true difference exists in the clinic utilization percentages of the freshmen and senior populations, we want to be able to detect that difference in our sample data. In evaluation, statistical power is directly related to sample size: Large samples have more power than small samples. Our goal therefore is to choose a sample size with sufficient power for future statistical significance tests.

There are no conventions for choosing a level of power. Cohen (1977, 1988) proposes that .80 power (or β = .20) is reasonable for general use. Lipsey (1998), however, argues that this implies that a Type I error is four times (4 × .05 = .20) more important than a Type II error. He recommends that if a Type II error is at least as important as a Type I error, α and β should have equal values. Thus, if α = .05, then power would equal .95 (1 – β = 1 – .05 = .95).

Similarly, we also may want to reduce α, or the probability of rejecting the null hypothesis when no difference between groups actually exists in the population. To do so, the same association applies: Smaller levels of α require larger sample sizes.

A final question remains to be answered: How big of a difference in the clinic utilization percentages between freshmen and seniors do we want to be able to detect? Suppose that 50% of the seniors visited the teen clinic at least once in the school year. Suppose that one member of the evaluation team speculates that 45% of the freshmen visited the clinic at least once in the past school year. To detect this 5-point difference (5 = 50 – 45), a sample size of 1,569 students would be required in *each* class (a requirement impossible to satisfy because the largest class size is 400 students). Now suppose that another member of the evaluation team thinks that only 30% of the freshmen visited the clinic. To detect this 20-point difference, a sample size of 108 students is required per class. In short, large samples are required to detect small differences, as shown in Table 7.3 (Dennis 1994).

These lessons have some important implications for the evaluation of the teen clinic. As described earlier, in the example in Step 1, let's suppose the freshman and senior classes each have 300 students, and utilization data are collected for 250 students in each class. With a fixed sample size, the central question becomes "How big of a difference in clinic utilization between the two groups can be detected with a sample size of 250 students per group?"

The answer to this question appears in Figure 7.2, which presents a *power chart* containing *effect sizes* (ES) for different sample sizes and power levels for an α = .05 two-tailed test or α = .025 one-tailed test. An effect size is the *minimum detectable difference* between the means of two groups for a given sample size, power, and α level. In our example, we want to find the minimum detectable difference between the utilization percentages (or proportions) for the two classes with a sample size of 250 students per group. To find the effect size, first locate the 250 sample size on the horizontal axis. Then, go up the vertical line for the 250 sample size and find where it meets the horizontal line for

TABLE 7.3   Smallest Detectable Outcome for Various Sample Sizes, Assuming Two
Groups, 80% Power, and 5% Type I Error Rate

Minimum Number Per Group	Percentage Point Differences $(P_2 - P_1)$	Correlation Coefficient
39,243	1-5	.01
9,810	1-5	.02
4,359	1-5	.03
2,452	1-5	.04
1,569	5	.05
1,089	5-10	.06
800	5-10	.07
612	5-10	.08
484	10	.09
392	10-15	.10
324	10-15	.11
272	10-15	.12
232	10-15	.13
200	15	.14
174	15-20	.15
152	15-20	.16
135	15-20	.18
120	15-20	.19
108	20	.20
97	20-25	.21
80	20-25	.23
68	25	.25
57	25-30	.27
49	30	.29
42	30-35	.31
38	35	.33
33	35-40	.35
30	40	.37
24	45	.41
18	50	.45
14	> 50	.49

SOURCE: Dennis ML. "Ethical and Practical Randomized Field Experiments." In: Wholey JS, Hatry HP, Newcomer KE, eds. *Handbook of Practical Program Evaluation*. San Francisco: Jossey Bass; 1994:168.

Figure 7.2. Power Chart for α = .05, Two-Tailed Test, or α = .025, One-Tailed Test

SOURCE: Lipsey MW. *Design Sensitivity: Statistical Power for Experimental Research.* © Copyright 1990 by Sage Publications, Inc. Reprinted by permission of Sage Publications, Inc.

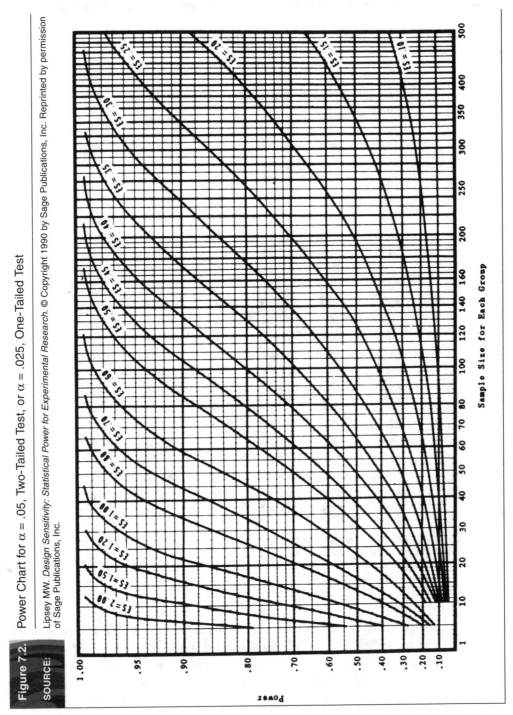

TABLE 7.4   Arcsine Transformation (Φ) for Proportions (ρ)

ρ	Φ	ρ	Φ	ρ	Φ	ρ	Φ
.01	.200	.26	1.070	.51	1.591	.76	2.118
.02	.284	.27	1.093	.52	1.611	.77	2.141
.03	.348	.28	1.115	.53	1.631	.78	2.165
.04	.403	.29	1.137	.54	1.651	.79	2.190
.05	.451	.30	1.159	.55	1.671	.80	2.214
.06	.495	.31	1.181	.56	1.691	.81	2.240
.07	.536	.32	1.203	.57	1.711	.82	2.265
.08	.574	.33	1.224	.58	1.731	.83	2.292
.09	.609	.34	1.245	.59	1.752	.84	2.319
.10	.644	.35	1.266	.60	1.772	.85	2.346
.11	.676	.36	1.287	.61	1.793	.86	2.375
.12	.707	.37	1.308	.62	1.813	.87	2.404
.13	.738	.38	1.328	.63	1.834	.88	2.434
.14	.767	.39	1.349	.64	1.855	.89	2.465
.15	.795	.40	1.369	.65	1.875	.90	2.498
.16	.823	.41	1.390	.66	1.897	.91	2.532
.17	.850	.42	1.410	.67	1.918	.92	2.568
.18	.876	.43	1.430	.68	1.939	.93	2.606
.19	.902	.44	1.451	.69	1.961	.94	2.647
.20	.927	.45	1.471	.70	1.982	.95	2.691
.21	.952	.46	1.491	.71	2.004	.96	2.739
.22	.976	.47	1.511	.72	2.026	.97	2.793
.23	1.000	.48	1.531	.73	2.049	.98	2.858
.24	1.024	.49	1.551	.74	2.071	.99	2.941
.25	1.047	.50	1.571	.75	2.094		

SOURCE: Lipsey MW. *Design Sensitivity: Statistical Power for Experimental Research.* © Copyright 1990 by Sage Publications, Inc. Reprinted by permission of Sage Publications, Inc.

power = .80. The two lines intersect on a curve labeled "ES = .25," indicating that the sample size is large enough to detect an effect size of .25.

To interpret the meaning of the .25 effect size, we can use the arcsine transformations of the proportions (or percentages) in Table 7.4. Again, let's assume that the proportion of seniors who used the clinic was .50, which has a corresponding arcsine value of 1.571 (see Table 7.4). Given a .25 effect size, the minimum proportion of freshmen using the clinic is defined by 1.571 − .250 = 1.321, which corresponds to a proportion of about .38. Thus, the .25 effect size indicates that a 12-point difference between the two groups (.12 = .50 − .38) is the smallest difference that can be detected with a sample size of 250 students per group for these α and power levels. This 12-point range is consistent with the 10-15 point range for a sample size of 250 in Table 7.3. If the actual difference between the population of freshmen and seniors turns out to be smaller, say 6 points rather than 12 points, the statistical test will *not* be significant with the 250 sample size for each group.

Effect sizes for continuous variables are calculated by dividing the difference between the means of the two groups by the pooled (or common) standard deviation of their distribution, as shown in the following equation:

$$ES = \text{(Mean of Group A − Mean of Group B)}/$$
$$\text{Pooled Standard Deviation}$$

The pooled standard deviation for the two groups can be estimated from sample data using the following formula (Lipsey 1990:78):

$$s = \sqrt{(S_a^2 + S_b^2)/2}$$

where S_a and S_b are the variances for the two groups. Once the effect size is calculated, the next step is to locate the relevant ES curve in Figure 7.2. After the curve is located, the power associated with different sample sizes per group can be identified readily by moving up and down the curve, and noting its intersections with the horizontal (power) and vertical (sample size) axes. If power calculations are based on a two-tailed test, as illustrated in Figure 7.2, future data analyses also should use two-tailed statistical tests for consistency.

Sample size and power also are critical issues for impact evaluations. If a program has an impact, a sample size with adequate power is required to detect it. Although different impact designs exist (see Chapter 4), there are only three basic ways to estimate program effects:

1. Comparing baseline and outcome scores for members of the treatment group, such as in the pretest-posttest design
2. Comparing outcomes in the treatment group with the outcomes of another group at a single point in time, such as in the posttest-only comparison group design or the posttest-only control group design

3. Comparing the change in outcomes in the treatment group with the change in outcomes in another group, such as in the pretest-posttest control group design or the nonequivalent comparison group design (Dennis 1994)

Power and minimum sample sizes for all three types of comparisons can be performed using the power chart and effect sizes in Figure 7.2. For example, we may want to estimate the effect of a health promotion program to increase regular exercise using a randomized, posttest-only control group design. Given a minimum effect size of .20, about 400 persons per group are required to detect this effect with power = .80 and α = .05 with a two-tailed test.

Alternatively, suppose we wanted to determine whether a 2-month continuing education class increased the knowledge of the health professionals using a nonequivalent comparison group design. The treatment group consists of health professionals who attended the class, and the comparison group consists of health professionals with the same credential who did not attend the class. Baseline and follow-up measures of knowledge are collected from the members of both groups, and the average change in knowledge is calculated in each group. Next, a minimum effect size is chosen based on the smallest *difference* between the average change score in the treatment group and the average change in the comparison group that the evaluation wants to be able to detect. Once the effect size is defined, the sample sizes for different power levels can be determined from Figure 7.2.

This raises an important question for impact evaluation: What effect size is a reasonable choice for estimating the minimum sample size required for an evaluation? Based on treatment effectiveness research in the behavioral sciences, Cohen (1977, 1988) proposed that a .20 effect size may be regarded as a small effect, .50 as a medium effect, and .80 as a large effect. More recently, Lipsey and Wilson (1993) examined the effect sizes reported in more than 300 psychological, behavioral, and education intervention studies. The median effect size was .44, with the 20th percentile at .24 and the 80th percentile at .68. This evidence suggests that .20 is a reasonable minimum effect size—large enough to be relevant but not so small that it may represent an extreme outcome for health programs (Lipsey 1998).

These methods for selecting a sample size are based on the simple comparison of means between two groups. In some impact evaluations, program effects are estimated using analysis of covariance, repeated measures, and other, more complex analytical techniques, and separate formulas for estimating effect size exist for these circumstances. Cohen (1977, 1988) provides a comprehensive set of formulas for calculating minimum sample sizes for a variety of evaluation designs. Kraemer and Thiemann (1987) also provide methods for estimating sample sizes based on the evaluation design's *critical effect size*; their methods take into account such factors as unequal sample sizes, repeated measures, and the type of statistical analysis when estimating minimum sample size requirements. For example, when estimating program impacts using a regression model, control variables may be included in the model to explain variation in the dependent variable. If a control variable accounts for only a small proportion of the variation in the dependent variable, the effect size changes little; however, if the control variable accounts for a large proportion of the variance, say 75%, the effect size doubles, which can greatly increase statistical power (Lipsey 1998).

In addition to textbooks, computer software also exists for conducting power calculations and estimating minimum sample size requirements. This software can aid evaluators in calculating minimum sample sizes (Lipsey 1998). In evaluations with complex designs and statistical analyses, a statistician should be consulted to derive minimum sample size requirements.

STEP 7: SELECT THE SAMPLE

If random or nonrandom sampling is necessary, and if the minimum sample size requirements are satisfied, the next step is to actually select the sample. On the other hand, if the minimum sample size requirements are not satisfied for answering an evaluation question, the evaluator may have to abandon answering the question or may be able to return to Act I and revise the question, employing qualitative methods for answering it with a small sample size.

DOCUMENT REVIEW EVALUATIONS

Some evaluations of program implementation do not entail the collection of information from people themselves (Patton 1987, 1990, 1997). For example, suppose a local health department and two social service agencies have formed a collaborative partnership to improve the coordination of services that they provide to homeless people, and an evaluation is conducted to assess the extent of collaboration in the partnership. Major sources of information for the evaluation are documents from the agencies, such as minutes from meetings, paper correspondence, e-mail correspondence, or financial transactions. Content analysis of program documents is a common qualitative method for developing a more in-depth understanding of the program's history and the extent of collaboration. The steps described in this chapter typically apply to this form of data collection only when eligibility criteria are imposed for selecting the documents (such as selecting documents only from a specific month in a year), or when documents are sampled in some way.

SUMMARY

The first steps in designing an evaluation of a health program are to define the target populations for answering each question of the evaluation and to specify the eligibility criteria that define who is included and excluded in each population. Once the eligible members in each target population are defined, a key issue is whether the size of the population is large enough to answer each evaluation question. If the size of the target population is large, members of the target population can be sampled using a random or nonrandom sampling design to reduce the time and cost of data collection. If the size of the target population is small, the program may have to be evaluated using qualitative methods that can be applied in small populations.

Once the target populations and samples are chosen, the next step is to define the measures that will be collected from them, which are the topics of the next chapter.

LIST OF TERMS _____

Adjunct population

Cluster sampling

Confirmatory/disconfirmatory sampling

Convenience sampling

Criterion sampling

Critical case sampling

Disproportionate stratified sampling

Effect size

Efficiency of sample design

Eligibility

Exclusion criteria

Extreme or deviant case sampling

Homogeneous groups sampling

Inclusion criteria

Maximum variation sampling

Minimum detectable difference

Participant recruitment tree

Post-stratification sampling

Precision

Probability sample designs

Proportionate stratified sampling

Purposive sample designs

Sampling error

Simple random sampling

Snowball/chain/network sampling
Statistical power
Systematic random
  sampling

Target population
Type I error
Type II error
Typical case sampling

_____STUDY QUESTIONS

1. An evaluation conducts a random sample of program participants and asks them to complete a questionnaire to assess their attitudes about the program. Does the evaluator need to be concerned about internal validity when conducting the survey?

2. What is the difference between random and nonrandom sampling designs? Is a random sampling design always better than a nonrandom design? In quantitative evaluations, do minimum sample size requirements apply to nonrandom sampling designs?

3. What is the difference between calculating a minimum sample size and calculating a minimum detectable difference?

4. An evaluator is conducting an impact evaluation using a posttest-only pre-experimental design. What should the evaluator do if the number of individuals in the intervention and comparison groups is too small to detect a meaningful difference between the two groups?

CHAPTER 8

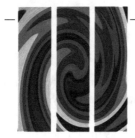

Measurement and Data Collection

Once the target populations and samples are selected, the next step in the evaluation process is to identify and collect information about each one to answer all the evaluation questions about the program. This is an important step in the evaluation process because the findings of the evaluation hinge directly on the type, amount, and quality of the information collected about the program and its target populations. When planning an evaluation, the goal is—to the extent possible—to identify *all* the information required to answer *all* of the questions *before* the information is collected. A great deal of careful and meticulous forethought is necessary to accomplish this goal. The payoffs of doing so come later in the evaluation process, when all the information to answer the questions is available for analysis, which, in turn, increases the likelihood that the evaluation questions actually will be answered, and that the results will be used in decision making.

The process of collecting information about the program depends on whether quantitative or qualitative methods (or both) are employed to answer the evaluation questions. Returning to the evaluation of the high school clinic introduced in Chapter 7, consider the following three questions asked about the clinic:

A: What percentage of students saw the clinic nurse or the mental health specialist at least once during the school year?

B: Are the utilization percentages similar or different across the four grades?

C. What are the reasons why students did not visit the clinic?

Questions A and B can be answered by collecting quantitative information about students in the high school. Quantitative evaluation usually assumes that programs are stable, observable, and measurable (Merriam 1998). Knowledge is created by breaking a program into its parts (such as the models of program theory and implementation in Chapter 3), using numbers to express or profile the parts, and then applying statistical analysis to examine the variation and relationships among the parts (Merriam 1998; Weiss 1998a). The answer to question A entails counting the number of students who did and did not visit the clinic in the school year. In question B, knowledge is gained through *deductive* reasoning—in this case, a statistical test providing definitive evidence that the percentage of students visiting the clinic is similar or different across grades.

In contrast, question C can be answered by collecting qualitative information from students who did not visit the clinic. Although quantitative methods create knowledge by breaking a program into its parts, qualitative methods build knowledge by revealing how the parts work together to form the program (Merriam 1998). In qualitative evaluation, the health program is viewed as a "lived experience," and knowledge is gained by understanding what this experience means to individuals in their own words (Merriam 1998; Patton 1997; Weiss 1998a). Although more than 40 types of qualitative methods exist (Tesch 1990), evaluators typically collect rich, detailed information about a program through focus groups, informal interviewing, observing program activities, reviewing program documents, or employing ethnographic and case study methods to achieve a deeper understanding of the program (Weiss 1998a). In question C, knowledge is gained through *inductive* reasoning, where detailed information is collected from students in focus groups (as described in Chapter 7) to derive or discover general themes, categories, typologies, hypotheses, or even theory, that explains why students did not visit the clinic (Merriam 1998).

Because data collection is fundamentally different for quantitative and qualitative evaluation, each is addressed in a separate section of this chapter. The first section addresses measurement and data collection methods for evaluation questions that require quantitative information to answer them, and the second section discusses collection issues for evaluation questions that require qualitative information to answer them.

MEASUREMENT AND DATA COLLECTION
IN QUANTITATIVE EVALUATIONS

The identification and collection of quantitative information to answer evaluation questions is a process composed of the following seven steps:

1. Decide what concepts to measure.
2. Identify measures of the concepts.
3. Assess the reliability, validity, and responsiveness of the measures.
4. Identify and assess the data source of each measure.
5. Choose the measures.
6. Organize the measures for data collection and analysis.
7. Collect the measures.

The section begins with a brief review of basic concepts and definitions in measurement and classification. Then each step of the process is reviewed in sequence.

The Basics of Measurement and Classification

All evaluation questions entail the measurement of concepts. To illustrate this point, let's draw from the Medicare demonstration described in Chapter 3, where one of the impact questions is to determine the effect of the package of preventive services on depression among older adults. To answer the impact question, information about depression must be collected for each adult in the demonstration. In this context, depression is a *concept*—that is, a dimension of health. The true depression in each adult cannot be observed directly. As a substitute, each adult is asked to complete the 20-item Center for Epidemiologic Studies Depression Scale (CES-D Scale), which is composed of 20 items capturing observable symptoms of depression (Radloff 1977). For each person who completes the scale, answers are summed according to a set of rules, and the possible range of scores is from 0 to 60, with higher scores indicating more depression symptoms. In short, the CES-D scale is the *operational definition* of the concept of depression for the impact evaluation (Blalock 1972).

The *measurement* of depression is the process of assigning a CES-D score, or number, to each adult according to the instructions and rules in its operational definition (Kaplan 1964). A *measure* is the specific CES-D score assigned to a specific adult, based on the person's responses to the 20-item scale and the rules for computing the CES-D score in the operational definition (Kaplan 1964). If the measures are identical for all adults, the CES-D score is called a *constant*. If the measures vary across adults, the CES-D score is called a *variable*. Measures that are constants or have very little variation typically have less value in health program evaluation, mainly because the goal of evaluation is to describe or explain variation in measures, and this goal does not apply to constants.

Measurement is the process of sorting and assigning numbers to people in quantitative evaluations. In qualitative evaluations, *classification* is a similar process for assigning people into a set of pigeonhole categories that have different names (Simon 1969). For example, the quantitative results from the CES-D scale may reveal that 14% of older adults have elevated depressive symptoms (Unutzer et al. 1997). Based on this finding, older adults with high CES-D scores are interviewed to identify the reasons for depression. If people report different reasons for their depression (e.g., the death of a family member, stress from a chronic illness, etc.), the reasons become a variable in the evaluation. Each reason is a category of the variable, and classification is the process of assigning each adult to one or more or the categories.

For simplicity, the term *measure* is used generically and applies to both measurement and classification in this chapter.

Step 1: Decide What Concepts to Measure

With this foundation of measurement and classification, the first step is to identify all the concepts that will be measured in the evaluation. This step is critically important for impact evaluations. If data collection begins in an impact design and someone discovers that a concept was overlooked, it is usually difficult to measure the omitted concept later on because the evaluation has a limited budget, the observation period is over, or for other reasons. In contrast, if a concept is overlooked in an implementation evaluation, or if a new concept is discovered in the course of data collection, implementation evaluations often have the flexibility to measure the concept *in some form* (as described later in Step 2) at a later date.

The best way to identify concepts is to list all the concepts in the evaluation's conceptual model (as described earlier in Chapter 3). For example, in the conceptual model for the Medicare demonstration in Figure 3.1, concepts are divided into different categories: individual characteristics, health risk, self-efficacy/autonomy, health status, and health service utilization and costs. *Each* individual characteristic and *each* health risk is a concept. Similarly, *each* dimension of self-efficacy, health status, health service utilization, and cost is a concept. In this step, the goal is simply to develop a list of the concepts and sort them into mutually exclusive categories, such as those shown in Figure 3.1.

If you spent much effort in Act I developing a comprehensive model containing most of the concepts for answering the evaluation questions, you will reap great dividends in this step of the measurement process. On the other hand, if the conceptual model of the health program is relatively simple and contains only some of the concepts for answering the evaluation questions, the model should be upgraded to portray most of or all the concepts for completing the evaluation.

Most conceptual models of health programs illustrate how the program and other factors produce expected outcomes. Health programs also may produce unexpected outcomes, either beneficial or harmful, that are not included in the program's conceptual model. The health literature, program staff, decision makers, and other evaluators may help identify unexpected outcomes and thereby ensure they are measured and examined in the evaluation.

Once a comprehensive list of concepts emerges, it may be apparent that the evaluation lacks sufficient time and resources to measure all of them. In this case, the list of concepts must be whittled down in some way. One method for paring the list is to organize the concepts into three groups: essential, moderately important, and optional. Essential concepts should always be retained, and optional concepts often can be discarded. Concepts that are moderately important should be discarded only when doing so does not jeopardize the integrity of the evaluation—that is, all the evaluation questions can still be answered, even if a moderately important concept is omitted. Another method for reducing the number of concepts is to rate the importance of each evaluation question and to eliminate those that are less important to decision makers.

Step 2: Identify Measures of the Concepts

Once all the concepts are identified and sorted into mutually exclusive categories, the next step is to identify one or more operational definitions, or measures, of each concept. In general, measures of concepts can be identified through three basic approaches:

1. Literature searches to identify published measures of concepts that can be used without modification

erature searches to identify published measures that can be modified to
.leasure a concept

Creation of measures from scratch

Health program evaluations typically use all three approaches to measure concepts.

Identify Published Measures

The first approach is to search the literature for published measures of each concept. A rich source of measures is published evaluations of similar health programs that answer similar kinds of questions about the program. For example, published evaluations about high school clinics may contain measures of clinic utilization that are well suited for an evaluation of a new clinic in a high school. Similarly, published evaluations of programs to increase the use of preventive services among older adults may contain measures of use of preventive services and health status, as well as factors that influence them.

One way to identify publications of health program evaluations is to perform a computer search of the relevant literature databases. Comprehensive citation indexes in health care are MEDLINE, which contains citations from more than 3,500 journals worldwide, and HealthSTAR, which contains citations focusing on the clinical and nonclinical aspects of health care delivery. In addition, because health program evaluations often measure concepts from different disciplines, citation indexes for those disciplines also are important sources of measures. For example, PsycINFO contains citations from psychological journals, ERIC contains citations from education journals, and the Social Science Index (which is part of the ISI Web of Science literature database) contains citations from journals in sociology, economics, anthropology, political science, social work, and other disciplines. After relevant publications are identified, their reference lists also may contain other relevant publications about similar program evaluations that were not identified in the computer literature search. These articles also should be examined for measures of concepts.

Another source of measures is books that contain an inventory of measures of common concepts in the health field. Over the past three decades, a vast literature has emerged containing literally hundreds of measures of health status, patient satisfaction, health service utilization and expenditure, health behavior, and other concepts. Books devoted to these measures appear at the end of this chapter. Similarly, Orwin et al. (1998), Scheirer (1981, 1994), Scheirer et al.

(1995), and Morris and Fitz-Gibbon (1978) describe measures of program implementation that have been used in previous evaluations.

Colleagues also are sources of published measures of concepts. For example, a professional specializing in health programs for teenagers may have an in-depth knowledge of published evaluations of high school clinics, as well as experience in using the measures in her or his own work. Knowledgeable colleagues also are useful for cross-checking the comprehensiveness of the computer literature search. If a colleague identifies the same publications that were uncovered in the literature search, the overlap provides evidence that the key articles and measures were detected in the literature search.

Another reason for searching for measures in the published literature is to increase your understanding of the properties of the measure. For example, a published evaluation of a high school clinic may contain descriptive statistics for the percentage of students who visited the clinic, the average number of times the students visited the clinic, and the percentage of students seeing each type of provider in the clinic. These descriptive statistics can help an evaluator judge the value of the measures and whether they are suitable measures for the proposed evaluation. In particular, measures that exhibit little variation, or that are highly correlated with other measures of the same concept, may have little value and might be safely dropped, especially if the time and cost of collecting them are high. In addition, published descriptive statistics often are valuable sources of information for calculating minimum sample size requirements, as described in Chapter 7. Finally, published statistics also can help decision makers, the evaluator, and other interest groups and individuals develop insights about what kind of results to expect in Act III of the evaluation process.

Last, when health programs are evaluated using the same measures, their findings can be compared more easily, which contributes to the cumulative knowledge of what programs do and do not work and the reasons why (Shortell and Richardson 1978).

Modify Published Measures

Sometimes an extensive literature search reveals no suitable published measures of a given concept. In this situation, the second approach is to modify a measure of a similar concept. For example, Grembowski et al. (1993) developed operational definitions and measures of an older adult's self-efficacy in performing five health behaviors: regular exercise, consuming less dietary fat, weight control, avoidance of heavy drinking, and not smoking. Another evaluation may want to measure participants' self-efficacy of performing a different health behavior, such as eating more fiber or flossing teeth regularly. The self-efficacy items for fiber consumption and tooth flossing could be developed by modifying the words in the published items. The advantage of this approach is that the new measure is based on a previous measure with known properties, such as its average, standard deviation, and, if available, its reliability and validity (which are discussed in the next section). The disadvantage is that once a measure is modified *in any way*, the modified measure is no longer comparable to the original measure. This is an insurmountable problem if a goal of the evaluation is to compare the findings based on the modified measure with the published findings from the original measure.

Create New Measures

If the first and second approaches do not identify a measure of a concept, the measure and its operational definition must be created from scratch. Sudman and Bradburn (1982), Aday (1996), and Salant and Dillman (1994) provide guidance for writing single-item questions for surveys. DeVellis (1991) provides guidelines for constructing multi-item scales, such as the CES-D scale. Because these scales take time and skill to construct, an evaluation should have both in ample supply before doing so. Time and funds permitting, reliability and validity assessments should be performed of new measures of key concepts in the evaluation, as described in Step 4.

Step 3: Assess the Reliability, Validity, and Responsiveness of the Measures

After one or more measures of the concepts are identified, the next step is to assess their reliability, validity, and responsiveness. The goal of measurement is to accurately measure an underlying concept. *Measurement error* is the amount of discrepancy between a measure and the true value of the concept, and the goal is to select measures that have the smallest amount of error. Reliability, validity, and responsiveness assessments are the mechanism for achieving this goal and are reviewed in this step.

Reliability Assessment

Two types of measurement error exist: random error and nonrandom error. *Reliability* is a source of *random measurement error* and is defined as the extent to which the *same measure* gives the same results on *repeated applications* (American Psychological Association 1985; Carmines and Zeller 1979; Gehlbach 1993; Shortell and Richardson 1978). For example, 100 adults are asked to complete the CES-D in the early morning and the late afternoon of the same day. An adult may respond to the CES-D differently between the two occasions for reasons unrelated to the underlying concept, depression. For example, an adult may try harder and feel more tired or anxious at one time than another, or may have more familiarity with the scale in the afternoon than in the morning. For these and other reasons, we can expect that the correlation (also known as a *reliability coefficient*) between the daytime and afternoon scores is less than perfect (that is, less than 1.0). Landis and Koch (1977) provide the following guidelines for interpreting the correlation, or strength of agreement, in reliability assessments.

Magnitude of Correlation	Strength of Agreement
.00-.20	Poor
.21-.40	Fair
.41-.60	Moderate
.61-.80	Substantial
.81-1.0	Almost perfect

These guidelines suggest that .61 is a *minimum* standard of reliability. Reliability coefficients calculated from measures collected in one population may not apply to other populations with different characteristics.

In general, the reliability of a measure can be assessed through one of four methods, as shown in Table 8.1 (Carmines and Zeller 1979; Shortell and Richardson 1978). The first row of the table captures measures about people that can be collected *indirectly* by observers or raters, such as when hygienists count the number of teeth with decay or fillings in a person's mouth. The second row captures measures that are collected *directly* from people, such as through questionnaires, interviews, or tests. For both methods, reliability can be assessed at the *same point in time* or at *different points in time*. The combinations of the two methods and the two points in time form the four cells in Table 8.1.

Cell A (upper left) captures *interrater* or *interobserver* reliability, or the correlation *between* different observers at the *same* point in time. Interobserver reliability is assessed, for example, when three hygienists count the number of decayed and filled teeth in the mouths of 20 adults on the same day. Interobserver reliability exists if the counts of decayed and filled teeth are highly correlated *across* the three hygienists.

Cell B (upper right) addresses *intrarater* or *intraobserver* reliability, or the correlation between the observations made by the *same* observer at *different* points in time. Intraobserver reliability is assessed, for example, when the same

TABLE 8.1   Summary of Reliability Assessment Methods

Measurement Method	Time Interval	
	Same Point in Time	Different Points in Time
Observers/raters	**A** Interrater or interobserver reliability; correlate judgments made by different observers at same point in time	**B** Intrarater and intraobserver reliability; correlate judgments made by the same person at two different points in time
Tests, questionnaires, and surveys	**C** Split-half reliability; internal consistency reliability	**D** Test-retest reliability; alternative-form reliability

SOURCE: Adapted from Shortell SM, Richardson WC. *Health Program Evaluation.* St. Louis, MO: Mosby Company; 1978:76.

hygienist counts the number of decayed and filled teeth in the mouths of 20 people, then repeats the same exercise with the same 20 people some time later (assuming that no new fillings were placed in the intervening time). Intraobserver reliability exists if the hygienist's counts at the different time points are highly correlated with each other.

Inter- and intrarater reliability assessments are commonly performed in qualitative evaluations (Morris and Fitz-Gibbon 1978). The goal of several qualitative techniques is to classify information into one or more categories. For example, content analysis of transcripts from focus groups, minutes from advisory board meetings, or other sources may be used to count the number of times that individuals mention specific topics or themes. Interrater reliability is assessed when two or more raters are conducting the content analyses at the same point in time, and the correlation between the counts of the raters is calculated. Intrarater reliability is assessed when one person counts the occurrences of each topic or theme, the same person repeats the exercise after a sufficient time has elapsed to reduce the influence of memory, and the correlation between the two assessments is calculated.

The second row of Table 8.1 refers to measures collected directly from people. Cell C (lower left) lists two methods for assessing the *reliability of a test or survey instrument* at the *same* point in time. The *split-half method* is well-suited for assessing the reliability of knowledge, health status, or other scales composed of multiple items. The items from the scale are randomly divided into two halves, which are completed by the same individuals at the same point in time. If the scale is reliable, there should be a high correlation between the scores of the two halves. For example, Radloff (1977) reports a split-reliability coefficient of .76 for the CES-D in a general population of Caucasians, which indicates "substantial" strength of agreement.

The second method is known as *internal consistency reliability*. The method can be used in two ways. In the first way, two questions that measure the same concept but with different wording are placed in different sections of a questionnaire, which is administered at a single point in time. If the items are reliable, the scores for the two items should be correlated strongly, or "internally consistent" with each other. The second way is designed to measure the internal consistency among the items in a scale administered at a point in time. Cronbach's alpha (Cronbach 1951) is the most popular method of estimating the intercorrelations among the items of the scale. In general, the value of alpha increases as the average correlation among the items increases and as the number of items in the scale increases (Carmines and Zeller 1979). Items cannot be added indefinitely to increase reliability, however, mainly because the gain in reliability declines with the addition of each item and because each additional item increases the time and resources to construct the scale. Continuing the previous example, Radloff (1977) obtained a Cronbach's alpha of .85 for the CES-D in the general, Caucasian population.

Cell D of Table 8.1 (lower right) presents two methods for assessing the *reliability of a test or survey instrument* at *different* points in time. *Test-retest reliability* refers to administering a scale, test, or questionnaire to the same people at different points in time. Nunnally (1972) advises that the test-retest be completed within 2 weeks to 1 month. The scale is reliable if a strong correlation exists between the scores of the same scale (or test or questionnaire) at the two points in time. One problem with this method is that reliability may be overestimated because of memory (Carmines and Zeller 1979). If the time interval between the two tests is relatively short, people will recall their earlier responses, and retest scores will be more consistent. For example, Radloff (1977) reports test-retest correlations for the CES-D ranging between .51 and .69 for time intervals ranging from 2 to 8 weeks, indicating a moderate strength of agreement.

This problem is overcome in the *alternative-form reliability method*, where two "alternative" forms of the *same* scale or questionnaire are administered to the *same* people at *different* points in time. In health program evaluation, short scales may be preferred over long scales because the former require less time for the respondent to complete. Therefore, when developing a scale, a long version and a short version of a scale may be developed to measure the same concept, and the goal is to administer the short form in the field *if* it is reliable—that is, it is highly correlated with the long form. Nunnally (1972) recommends that the two scales be administered 2 weeks apart to reduce the influence of memory and to allow day-to-day fluctuations in people to occur. As an example of the method, Shrout and Yager (1989) compared the 20-item CES-D with a shorter, 5-item version of the CES-D and found Cronbach's alpha of .59 and .64 in community and patient samples, respectively.

In summary, reliability addresses whether results are consistent across repeated measurements (Carmines and Zeller 1979). The more consistent the results across repeated measurements, the greater the reliability of the measure, and vice versa. Different methods exist for assessing the reliability of a measure, depending on the type of measure, whether the measure is administered through questionnaires or tests, or whether observers or raters are used to measure a concept. Because health program evaluations typically employ a variety of measures, different methods usually are required to assess their reliability. The reliability of each measure can be assessed by reviewing published reliability assessments in the literature or by actually conducting the reliability assessment in the context of the program. If the reliability of key measures of the evaluation is unknown, adequate time and resources should be built into the evaluation to perform the reliability assessments before data collection begins.

Validity Assessment

Measurement validity is the extent to which a measure actually measures what it is supposed to measure rather than some other concept (American Psychological Association 1985; Carmines and Zeller 1979; Gehlbach 1993; Shortell and Richardson 1978). For example, we might claim that mortality (dead vs. alive), being hospitalized overnight, and the number of days spent in bed at home because of illness or injury are valid or accurate measures of a person's "health status," but the measures are probably not valid for other purposes, such as measuring a person's knowledge of mathematics. The validity of a measure is influenced by *nonrandom measurement error*, which occurs when a measure is *systematically* higher or lower than the true score. For example, a program may be developed to improve the quality of care for patients with hypertension, and age-adjusted blood pressure is the program's measure of hypertension. Let's suppose the sphygmomanometer (or blood pressure gauge) malfunctions, and the blood pressure reading of each patient is 20 points higher than the true pressure. Because the readings are consistently high for all patients, we have evidence that nonrandom measurement error has influenced the measurement of each patient's actual blood pressure.

There are two key points to remember about measurement validity. First, *measurement* validity has a *different* meaning from *internal* validity, *external* validity, and *statistical conclusion* validity. Measurement validity refers to the accuracy of the measure of some underlying concept, and the term applies to both impact and implementation evaluations. Internal validity, external validity, and statistical conclusion validity are terms that apply to impact evaluations: Internal validity refers to the accuracy of the causal inferences from an impact design, external validity refers to the accuracy of the generalizations made from an impact design, and statistical conclusion validity refers to the accuracy of one's conclusions from a statistical test, as described in Chapter 4. Thus, although accuracy is the underlying concern in all these uses of the term *validity*, measurement validity is not the same thing as internal, external, or statistical conclusion validity.

The second key point is that reliability is a necessary, but not sufficient, condition for validity (Shortell and Richardson 1978). If 10 student nurses measure a person's blood pressure and obtain readings that range from 110/70 to 145/90 mmHg, the measure is not reliable, and therefore one can say little about the measure's potential validity (Gehlbach 1993; Shortell and Richardson 1978). On the other hand, a concept may be measured reliably but not be considered a valid measure of a given concept. For example, all 10 student nurses might reliably obtain a blood pressure reading of 145/95 mmHg, but if the blood pressure gauge malfunctions, the readings are invalid (Gehlbach 1993). As an alternative example, days absent from school might be measured reliably, but the absenteeism may not be a valid measure of the children's health status because children may be absent for a variety of reasons unrelated to health, such as family vacations and trips or observance of religious holidays (Shortell and Richardson 1978). In summary, a valid measure must by definition be reliable, but a reliable measure will not necessarily be a valid measure (Shortell and Richardson 1978).

In program evaluation, the goal is to select valid measures of concepts; therefore, the fundamental task is to obtain evidence about the validity of each measure from the published literature, from your own validity assessments, or from other sources. Unlike reliability assessment, validity is not measured directly but rather is assessed by comparing the measure with the purpose for which it is being used (Carmines and Zeller 1979). There are four major types and methods for assessing validity: *face* validity, *content* validity, *criterion* validity, and *construct* validity (American Psychological Association 1985; Carmines and Zeller 1979; Shortell and Richardson 1978).

Face validity refers to the common acceptance or belief that a measure indeed measures what it is supposed to measure. For example, most people would agree that mortality (dead vs. alive) is a valid measure of health status for patients undergoing cardiovascular surgery. Face validity is the weakest of the four types because the assessment is not supported by any evidence.

Content validity depends on the extent to which a measure contains a reasonable sample of the behaviors or attributes of a concept. This form of validity assessment typically is performed by assembling a panel of qualified judges who identify *all* the behaviors or attributes of a concept, select the sample of behaviors or attributes that are included in the measure, and assess whether the contents of the measure are representative of the larger concept. Content validity exists if the amount of agreement among the judges is high.

For example, the Rand-UCLA Health Services Utilization Study convened three panels, each composed of nine physicians, to rate, or measure, the "appropriateness" of indications for performing six medical and surgical procedures (Chassin et al. 1989). A comprehensive list of indications for each procedure was developed by reviewing the literature to identify all factors that physicians ordinarily take into account in their treatment recommendations to patients. Panelists were asked to rate the appropriateness of performing the procedure for each indication on a 1-to-9 scale, where "1" was *extremely inappropriate* and "9" was *extremely appropriate*. An "appropriate" indication meant that the expected health benefit (such as increased life expectancy or relief of pain) exceeded the expected negative consequences (such as mortality, morbidity, or pain produced by the procedure). An indication was defined as an "appropriate" reason for performing a procedure if the median rating was between 7 and 9 without disagreement, whereas an indication was defined as "inappropriate" if the median rating was between 1 and 3 without disagreement. An indication was defined as "equivocal" if the median rating was between 4 and 6 or if panelists disagreed on the appropriateness of performing the procedure for a specific indication. Given this operational definition of appropriate, equivocal, and inappropriate indications for performing a medical or surgical procedure, the indications were compared with clinical records from selected hospitals to measure the appropriateness of specific procedures performed in hospitals.

Criterion validity is assessed by comparing one measure with one or more other measures, or criteria. A measure has criterion validity if it is correlated highly with one or more of the criterion measures. The value of this evidence hinges greatly on the relevance of the criterion measure that is used (American Psychological Association 1985). Two types of criterion validity exist, *predictive* and *concurrent*. As its name implies, predictive validity assesses whether a measure accurately predicts the scores of the criterion measure in the future. Concurrent validity does the same thing, but both measures are collected at the same point in time. Concurrent validity is the preferable form for assessing measures of health status and scales created to measure a specific concept at a point in time. For example, Radloff (1977) reports that CES-D scores were correlated strongly with the criterion measures, which in this case were other depression scales.

Construct validity exists when a specific measure of a concept is associated with one or more other measures in a manner consistent with theoretically derived hypotheses (Carmines and Zeller 1979). For example, self-efficacy is an important concept in the conceptual model for the Medicare demonstration (see Figure 3.1). The concept of self-efficacy consists of two dimensions, efficacy expectations and outcome expectations. Based on the theory of self-efficacy and the demonstration's conceptual model, we might posit that (a) efficacy expectations and outcome expectations are correlated positively with each other and (b) that the correlation between efficacy and outcome expectations is larger than their correlation with other concepts, such as age, gender, or socioeconomic status. Findings from the Medicare demonstration are consistent with these hypotheses, although the sizes of the correlation were relatively small (Grembowski et al. 1993). In short, evidence of construct validity exists when measures of the *same* concept (in this case, efficacy expectations and outcome expectations) are correlated with each other but are *not correlated* with *different* concepts in the program's conceptual model (American Psychological Association 1985). On the other hand, if a measure is not associated with one or more similar concepts as hypothesized in the program's conceptual model, the usual inference is that the measure does *not* represent the underlying concept, and we conclude that the measure lacks construct validity *for that particular concept* (Carmines and Zeller 1979).

In summary, measurement validity refers to the extent to which a measure actually measures what it purports to measure. Different methods exist for assessing validity. In some cases, face validity may be adequate evidence of the accuracy of a measure. For example, the cost per unit of output is a commonly accepted measure of program efficiency (Shortell and Richardson 1978). In other cases, evidence of content, criterion, or construct validity is required, such as when an evaluation is using a new measure or trying to measure ill-defined concepts (Shortell and Richardson 1978).

The validity of each measure can be assessed by reviewing published validity assessments in the literature. If the program's target population is different from the publication's population, the published findings may not apply to the program evaluation. For example, Hayes and Baker (1998) found significant differences in reliability and validity of the English and Spanish versions of a patient satisfaction scale. If published reliability and validity assessments that match the evaluation's target population cannot be found, or published validity assessments do not exist for the key measures of the evaluation, adequate time and resources should be built into the evaluation to perform the validity assessments before data collection begins.

Responsiveness Assessment

As interest has grown in measuring the health outcomes of programs, so has concern about the *responsiveness* of health status measures. Responsiveness is the ability of a health status measure to detect small but important changes (Guyatt et al. 1987; Patrick and Erickson 1993). To illustrate this criterion of measurement, suppose that a health program is implemented to improve the physical function of adults with rheumatoid arthritis. The impacts of the program are estimated using a randomized design, and health outcomes are measured with a physical function scale. Let's assume the program actually increased physical functioning of the adults in the treatment group. For the scale to be responsive, we would expect the scores to be stable among adults in the control group and changing in the expected direction among adults in the treatment group. Different methods of assessing responsiveness exist, but the most common is to compare instrument scores before and after a treatment that is known to be efficacious (Deyo et al. 1991; Patrick and Erickson 1993). The evidence indicates that disease-specific measures are more responsive than global measures of health status, and evaluations commonly employ both types of measures to estimate the health impacts of programs or services. In summary, if health status is a key outcome of an impact evaluation, evidence also should be collected to assess the responsiveness of the measure.

Selection of Reliable, Valid, and Responsive Measures

Once evidence is gathered about the reliability, validity, and responsiveness (if applicable) of the alternative measures of each concept, it is time to select measures with the least amount of measurement error. The following guidelines are offered for measurement selection:

1. If a single measure of a concept is identified, the measure is acceptable *if* published evidence supports the reliability and validity of the measure. Similarly, if a new measure of a concept is created, the new measure is ac-

ceptable *if* original assessments indicate the measure has acceptable reliability and validity.

2. When two or more alternative measures of a concept exist, and the published evidence indicates that one measure has acceptable and greater levels of reliability and validity than the other measures, the more reliable and valid measure is the appropriate choice.

3. For measures of health status, published or original evidence also must support the responsiveness of the measure.

4. If two or more measures have similar, acceptable levels of reliability and validity, the choice typically is based on other factors, such as the measure's fit with the program objectives and the evaluation design, whether the measure captures potential unintended consequences of the program, the time and cost of data collection, ease of administration, characteristics of the target population (such as handicapping condition, native language, and ethnicity), and burden on respondents (American Psychological Association 1985; Neuhauser and Yin 1991).

5. If published or original evidence of the reliability and validity of a previous or new measure of a *key* concept does not exist, it may be advisable to not answer the question(s) that the measure addresses. This is particularly the case if the measure addresses a key outcome, program impacts are expected to be small, and the political stakes are high (Shortell and Richardson 1978).

Step 4: Identify and Assess the Data Source of Each Measure

Types of Data Sources

The next step is to identify and assess the source of data for *each* reliable and valid measure identified in Step 2. Because health program evaluations typically measure a variety of concepts, data often must be collected from a variety of sources. Table 8.2 lists common sources of data in health program evaluation (Fink 1993; Shortell and Richardson 1978). In general, two basic sources of data exist, *primary data sources* and *secondary data sources*. Primary (or "original") sources entail the collection of information directly from people. Examples include the different types of survey techniques, the collection of clinical measures from patients, and the observation of people's behavior or characteristics. Secondary (or "existing" or "precollected") sources refer to existing,

TABLE 8.2   Common Data Sources in Health Program Evaluation

Original or "primary" data sources

    Physical examinations

    Self-administered surveys

    Personal or telephone surveys

    Health knowledge tests

    Self-administered diaries for recording personal behavior

    Achievement tests, such as the ability to perform CPR

    Observations such as time and motion studies, ethnography, or counting decayed teeth in people's mouths

Existing or "secondary" data sources

    Medical records, such as patient charts and case management files

    Vital statistics, such as birth and death certificates

    National data sets, such as the National Health Interview Survey

    Public/private insurance claims

    Hospital discharge databases

    Databases of professional associations

historical data about the program. Program records and agency files are natural sources of secondary data, and common types of secondary data for health program evaluation include medical charts, health insurance claims, and birth and death certificates.

Advantages and Disadvantages of Primary and Secondary Data

The major advantage of primary data sources is that collecting information directly from people is often the only way to measure specific concepts, such as health attitudes and knowledge, health behavior, health status, or satisfaction with health care. Furthermore, in implementation evaluations, primary data sources, such as in-depth interviews with program clients and staff, are often critical for understanding "what goes on" within a health program.

The flip side of the coin is that secondary data usually take less time and costs less to collect than primary data, which is a major advantage for evaluations that must be completed quickly with limited funds. Secondary data also are ideal for implementation evaluations where concepts can be measured with secondary data, for impact evaluations with time series designs, and for designs with pretest and posttest observations (Shortell and Richardson 1978).

Secondary data may be used to measure concepts *if* their quality is acceptable. The major threats to the quality of secondary data are *incompleteness, inaccuracy, invalidity,* and *inconsistency* (Shortell and Richardson 1978). Previous studies have shown that health insurance claims may be incomplete—that is, claims may not exist in a database for all the health services that a person receives (Luft 1986). For example, Medicare fee-for-service claims are a common secondary data source for measuring the health services utilization and charges for older adults; however, people aged 65 and over also receive care from the Veterans Administration, health maintenance organizations, and other health agencies. The Medicare fee-for-service claims database therefore is an incomplete source of secondary data for these people.

Even if data are complete, they may be inaccurate as a result of errors in data entry or data processing or for other reasons, or the data may be invalid (Shortell and Richardson 1978). For example, a health clinic may have records of broken appointments that are complete and accurate, but the records are likely an invalid measure of patient satisfaction. Missed appointments may occur for a variety of reasons, such as problems with child care and transportation, that are unrelated to patient satisfaction with clinic services.

Finally, the quality of secondary data may be threatened by consistency problems, which have two common forms (Shortell and Richardson 1978). First, when a health program is implemented in several sites by multiple agencies, the different agencies may measure concepts in different ways. As a consequence, the secondary data across the sites are inconsistent and therefore cannot be used to compare performance across sites. Second, consistency problems also occur when the agency collecting the secondary data changes the definitions of the measures or how the measures are collected during the course of the program. For impact evaluations collecting pre- and postprogram secondary data, these changes are instrumentation threats to internal validity and undermine causal inferences about the program.

Factors Influencing the Choice of Data Sources

For some measures, a single data source can be identified readily based on the reliability and validity assessments in the previous step. For other measures,

TABLE 8.3   Relationship Between the Type of Data Source and the Type of Evaluation Design

	Type of Data Source	
Type of Evaluation Design	*Primary Data Sources*	*Secondary Data Sources*
Retrospective	A Feasible in some evaluation designs except those collecting preprogram data	B Essential for conducting the evaluation if data quality is acceptable
Cross-sectional or prospective	C Essential for point-in-time measures of people's knowledge, attitudes, behavior, or health status	D Preferable to primary sources if the quality of secondary data sources is acceptable

both primary or secondary data sources may exist. In this case, how does one choose between them? The following factors often influence these choices.

First, the type of evaluation design may influence the selection of data sources, as shown in Table 8.3. Retrospective evaluations may draw from both secondary and primary data sources. For example, retrospective evaluations of program implementation may interview the staff who administered the program at any time in the past year (cell A, upper left). In many retrospective evaluations, secondary data with acceptable quality are essential for measuring the program's performance in the past (cell B, upper right).

Similarly, cross-sectional and prospective evaluations also may employ both types of data sources. For example, in the Medicare demonstration, a prospective, randomized, pretest-posttest design was employed to estimate the program's effect on changes in self-efficacy, health behavior, health status, cost, and utilization. Because no secondary data sources exist for the self-efficacy, health behavior, and health status measures, primary data sources—in this case, both mail questionnaires and telephone interviews—are essential for measuring these concepts (cell C, lower left). Because Group Health Cooperative's information systems regularly collected cost and utilization information, those measures are collected through this secondary data source (cell D, lower right). Although the information system contains data for *all* older adults in the evaluation, the survey data exist only for adults who complete the survey. Thus, complete data for all measures exist only for those adults who completed all surveys across all time points in the evaluation design.

Second, primary and secondary data *must* be collected in an ethical manner that protects the rights of human subjects. For primary data collection, this means people who are asked for information must be informed fully about the evaluation. People must be informed explicitly that their participation is voluntary, that they are free not to answer any questions, and that refusal to participate or not answer specific questions will have no adverse consequences. Similarly, some secondary data resources, such as medical charts, require the written consent from the people who are asked to participate in the evaluation. Clearly, the requirements of informed consent are an important factor influencing the choice of data sources in virtually all evaluations. If either primary or secondary data sources may be selected to measure a concept, the choice may hinge on the feasibility of obtaining the informed consent from people in each mode of data collection.

Third, the choice of secondary versus primary data sources may be influenced by the *context* of the program, such as the characteristics of the target population, the burden that a mode of data collection imposes on people, whether the evaluation has qualified personnel to collect and analyze the data, whether evaluation staff have the technical skills to assess the reliability and validity of new measures and data sources, whether the evaluation team has access to secondary data sources, and other factors (Fink 1993; Weiss 1998a). For example, it may be extremely difficult to collect valid and reliable information from program participants if members of the evaluation team speak a language different from that of the program participants and if no previous questionnaires or scales exist in the native language of the program participants. In this case, measures from primary data sources may have to be abandoned and the evaluation confined to measures that can be obtained from secondary data sources.

A related concern is the burden placed on respondents. If the number of measures from primary data sources is large, the data collection demands imposed on people become excessive, which ultimately will lower the percentage of people consenting to participate in the evaluation. In this case, the burden of primary data collection can be reduced by collecting some of the measures from secondary data sources, which usually impose fewer burdens on people, if quality secondary data are available.

Before choosing either a primary or a secondary data source, a key issue to consider is whether the evaluation has access to the secondary data. When an evaluation team enters Act II of the evaluation process, it may assume that it will have access to secondary data upon request. Agencies, however, often have strong policies about releasing their data to outside parties, and some agencies may refuse to release *any* information to an evaluation team, particularly if the agency believes—for whatever reasons—that the results of the evaluation might portray the agency unfavorably. In short, an evaluation team always should obtain written permission to access secondary data sources that belong to outside agencies before data collection begins.

Finally, published evidence may indicate the advantages and disadvantages of measuring a concept using primary versus secondary data, providing evidence for selecting one mode over the other. For example, Brown and Adams (1992) examined the reliability and validity of patient reports of events in medical encounters (such as whether a blood pressure check, chest radiograph, mammogram, or electrocardiogram was performed) by comparing patient reports in telephone interviews with medical records. Findings indicate that patients generally are reliable reporters for a majority of the medical procedures addressed in the interview.

In summary, secondary data are less costly and time-consuming to collect than primary data. If secondary data are available and have acceptable quality, secondary data may be preferred over primary data sources, particularly if the evaluation must be performed in a short amount of time with limited funds (Shortell and Richardson 1978). On the other hand, primary data are recommended if the concept cannot be measured using secondary data, if secondary data are not available, or if secondary data exist but have quality problems. The choice of data sources also is influenced by other factors, such as the type of evaluation design and the features of the evaluation itself. If alternative measures and data sources exist for a given concept, data source selections are made by carefully weighing the advantages and disadvantages of each data source for each measure. Published evidence that compares the merits of alternative data sources is critical in making these assessments.

Step 5: Choose the Measures

After weighing the reliability and validity of the measures and the advantages and disadvantages of primary and secondary data sources, the next step is to select one or more measures and their respective data sources. If an evaluation is being performed by more than one evaluator, all members of the team should agree on the measures and data sources for all the concepts of the evaluation before data collection begins. In some evaluations, decision makers also are included in measurement and data source selection, which increases the likelihood that the results will actually be used in decision making in Act III of the evaluation process.

Step 6: Organize the Measures for
Data Collection and Analysis

Once the measures are selected, the next step is to sort them into categories that will organize the data analysis in the next chapter. This step has two parts.

The first part is to label each measure as either a *dependent variable*, an *independent* (or control) *variable*, or a *program* (or treatment) *variable*. The dependent variables of most programs are defined by the evaluation questions created in Act I of the evaluation process. For example, consider the evaluation question "Are patients satisfied with the program?" Patient satisfaction is the dependent variable, and the goal is to measure the *variation* in satisfaction among the patients in the program.

Now, consider a second question: "What factors influence patient satisfaction?" Patient satisfaction is still the dependent variable, and the goal is to identify factors—or independent variables—that explain the variation in patient satisfaction. A phrase such as "patient satisfaction *depends on* a patient's age, gender, and years of education" often helps to distinguish the dependent variable from the independent variables.

Finally, program variables are defined only for impact evaluations with treatment and control groups. The purpose of the program variable is to indicate whether a person is a member of the treatment group or the control group. For statistical reasons, a program variable usually has two values, 0 and 1, where 1 indicates a person is a member of the treatment group and 0 indicates the person is a member of the control group.

The second part is to categorize each measure by its *level of measurement*. Sorting the measures by their level of measurement is important because the different levels of measurement entail different forms of statistical and qualitative analyses (discussed in the next chapter). The four levels of measurement are *nominal, ordinal, interval* (or *categorical*), and *ratio*. Nominal measures are those that classify objects or events into two or more mutually exclusive categories. Gender (male vs. female), mortality (dead vs. alive), and program variables (treatment group vs. control group) are examples of nominal measures.

Ordinal measures are those that classify objects or events by the amount of a specific characteristic, but the differences between the categories cannot be measured on a constant scale. For example, a person may rate his or her health as either "excellent," "very good," "good," "fair," or "poor." The measure has an order; we know that excellent is better than very good, and that very good is better than good. The differences between each pair of categories, however, are not the same. That is, it is impossible to tell whether the difference between

TABLE 8.4   Documentation of Evaluation Measures: An Example From the Medicare Demonstration

Concept and Measure	Reference	Level of Measurement	Data Source/ Collection Method	When Collected
Health status				
Self-rated health	Adams and Benson 1990	Ordinal	Mail survey	Baseline and all follow-ups
Quality of Well-Being Scale	Kaplan et al. 1976	Ratio	Telephone interview	Baseline and all follow-ups
Health behavior/risk				
Exercise	Buchner et al. 1991	Nominal	Mail survey	Baseline and all follow-ups
Dietary fat	Kristal et al. 1990	Nominal	Mail survey	Baseline and all follow-ups
Personal characteristics				
Birth date (age)	Adams and Benson 1990	Ratio	Mail survey	Baseline only
Marital status	Adams and Benson 1990	Nominal	Mail survey	Baseline and all follow-ups

"excellent" and "very good" is identical to the difference between "fair" and "poor."

Interval measures are those that classify objects or events by the amount of a specific characteristic, and in addition the difference between observations can be measured on a scale that has no true zero point. For example, the difference between 3 and 5 is the same as the difference between 6 and 8. The Fahrenheit temperature scale and the CES-D depression scale are examples of interval measures. The advantage of interval measures is that they can be added or subtracted, but without a zero point they cannot be multiplied or divided.

Ratio measures are interval measures with a true zero point. Examples include measures of a person's annual income, the number of doctor visits in a given year, and the number of days spent in bed due to illness in the past 2 weeks. With a true zero point, ratio measures can be added, subtracted, multiplied, and divided.

Once the measures, the data sources, and their classifications are known, a table should be constructed documenting this information for all the measures in the evaluation. An example is presented in Table 8.4, which describes a small number of the measures in the Medicare demonstration. After the table is completed, all members of the evaluation team should review its contents to cross-check that no important measures were overlooked and that everyone approves the measures of the concepts. This agreement is vital in an evaluation, because after data collection begins, it is often too late to make major changes in the evaluation's measures.

Step 7: Collect the Measures

The final step is to actually collect the measures. Health program evaluations typically employ a wide variety of data collection methods, which are described in detail in several book and journal publications. At the end of this chapter, references on survey and health services research methods are presented for those seeking more in-depth information and guidance on these topics. Although references are always valuable, experience with a given data collection technique is often essential for the successful completion of data collection in the field. Evaluation teams therefore should be composed of members or consultants who have past experience with the data collection methods to guide the design and implementation of data collection.

DATA COLLECTION IN QUALITATIVE EVALUATION

In health program evaluation, two types of qualitative data collection can be defined, *informal* and *formal*. Informal data collection is an inevitable part of all health program evaluations—quantitative and qualitative—and occurs as a by-product of the evaluator's exposure to the program. That is, in designing an evaluation of an existing program, the evaluator's immediate task is to learn quickly about "what goes on" in the program through conversations with clients and staff, reviews of program documents, tours of program facilities, and other mechanisms. This informal data collection typically is not an explicit part of the evaluation's data collection plan but provides essential background information for understanding the underlying "culture" of the program, such as its social climate, the values and beliefs that staff bring to the program, or the agency's "commitment" to the program. This information is important because it provides "texture" and helps the evaluator understand the social reality in which the program operates, which, in turn, later helps the evaluator interpret the results from the more formal data analyses (Weiss 1998a).

For example, suppose that an evaluator is designing an impact evaluation of a series of health education classes the next time they are offered by a community clinic serving a diverse community. To plan the evaluation, the evaluator decides to observe one of the classes. Upon entering the room, the evaluator is immediately collecting informal data about the class: Is the class held in the basement or in a well-lighted room with windows? Do students sit in rows or in a circle? Are students in the room quiet or talking to each other? Are the students talking informally with the instructor before the class starts? What is the racial or ethnic background of the instructor, and how does it compare with the mix of racial or ethnic backgrounds of the students? The evaluator arranges a meeting with the instructor to learn more about the contents of the curriculum (that is, the intervention of the impact evaluation), and in the course of their conversations the evaluator learns that the class has attendance problems, but those who do attend are enthusiastic supporters of the class.

In short, virtually all evaluations of health programs occur in a social or cultural context, and informal data collection is a mechanism for grasping and understanding this context. When either planning or conducting evaluations of program impacts or implementation, evaluators should always be "on the lookout" for informal data collection opportunities.

Formal data collection consists of the planned collection of qualitative information that is designed specifically to answer one or more questions about the program. A wide variety of qualitative methods exist; Tesch (1990) lists 45 qualitative research methods, some overlapping with each other, that could be applied to the evaluation of health programs. Although detailed descriptions of these qualitative methods are beyond this textbook, Weiss (1998a) presents six qualitative methods of data collection that are common in the evaluation of social, health, and education programs. These methods can be used individually or in combination with each other. More detailed information about these and other qualitative methods can be found in the references at the end of this chapter.

> ▶ *Ethnography* is a descriptive method developed by anthropologists to study a culture, whether the culture is an African village or an emergency room (ER) of a hospital (Fetterman 1998). Ethnography entails intensive, long-term fieldwork. The ethnographer becomes a member of

the group, participating fully in daily activities, and over time absorbs the group's norms and values. The commitment must be long term for the ethnographer to be accepted and trusted by the group, and to cultivate close relationships with individuals, or "informants," who can provide specific information about the culture's norms, rituals, and other aspects of daily life. Through immersion in the culture, ethnographers may come to identify with the people they are studying, which can affect their objectivity. Returning to the ER example, to evaluate an intervention to improve the health outcomes and satisfaction of ER patients, an evaluator-ethnographer might become an ER employee to experience the ER's culture at first hand, absorb its norms and views, and understand how the intervention operates in its culture.

▶ *Participant-observation* is similar to ethnography but is typically less intensive and can be either short or long term. The evaluator participates in the program's activities, but the top priority is the detached observation of program activity and events on a day-to-day basis. By playing a role in the program, the evaluator comes to understand how the program works through both experience and observation.

▶ *Observation* is fieldwork where the evaluator visits the program's sites and makes careful, detailed observations about the program, with the goal of describing activities and understanding what they mean to program participants. Typically, observation occurs with full disclosure; everyone in the program knows who the evaluator is and what he is up to. The evaluator does not take part in program activities and therefore is less likely to influence the program than the ethnographer or participant-observer. For example, to evaluate a new health education curriculum in several high schools, an evaluator might spend several days—if not weeks or months—sitting in the health education classrooms of the high schools and observing what is taught, teacher-student interaction, and other aspects of the curriculum.

▶ *Informal interviewing* is an open-ended conversation, with a goal of understanding the program from the respondent's perspective. When interviewing people who run a program, the evaluator typically asks everyone one to three "core" questions about the program with the intention of comparing responses in the data analysis. Otherwise, different questions are asked to different people, because people have different knowledge about the program. The interview is conversational, with the evaluator using open-ended questions to pursue a topic, then probing to obtain in-depth information when necessary. The interviews continue until the evaluator reaches "closure" and has attained a full understanding of what goes on in the program.

▸ *Focus groups*, which have been mentioned in previous chapters, are a form of "group data collection" in which the evaluator assembles a group of 8-12 people around a table, asks them a question, and records their individual responses and the cross-talk between members of the group (Stewart and Shamdasani 1998). Focus groups are useful when the evaluator believes that more valuable information can be obtained through the group's conversations than can be gleaned through informal interviews with individuals, which are better suited for collecting information about individuals' attitudes, beliefs, or knowledge about the program. For example, to understand a health program, an evaluator might collect information from program staff through informal interviews but use focus groups to collect information from the program's participants.

▸ *Documents* from programs include laws, regulations, proposals for funding, budgets, correspondence, minutes from meetings, brochures, reports, slide presentations, newspaper clippings about the program, medical records, insurance claims, program Web sites, and so forth. Documents can provide a comprehensive portrait of program goals, objectives, and activities, and information gleaned from them can be used to cross-check the responses from program staff in informal interviews. Documents can be sources of quantitative information (such as the number of physician visits recorded in a medical chart) as well as qualitative information (for example, in a program administered through a three-agency collaborative partnership, the "strength" of the partnership is assessed through a content analysis of correspondence and minutes from meetings).

All these methods require fieldwork and extensive note-taking or other forms of data collection. A vast amount of text information can be collected, and schemes must be devised for organizing the information to facilitate later analysis. For example, Lofland and Lofland (1984) suggest sorting field notes into the following three files: (a) mundane files containing basic information about the program's sites, staff, activities, and so forth; (b) analytical files containing information that is central to answering the evaluation's questions, such as information about adherence to program protocols, unintended outcomes, or emerging themes expressed in individual interviews and focus groups; and (c) fieldwork files containing information about the process and problems of the fieldwork itself, such as the method for gaining entry into a program site, the method for selecting people to interview, and problems with observer bias. Just like quantitative evaluation, experience with a given qualitative method is often essential for the successful completion of data collection in the field; therefore, if the formal collection of qualitative information is planned, the evaluation team should be composed of members or consultants who have past experience with the method(s) to guide the design and implementation of the data.

Health programs are often complex, involving multiple and sometimes contradictory objectives with a large number and diversity of personnel (Shortell 1984). To handle the complexity and fully answer each question about a health program, evaluations often plan at the outset to collect both quantitative and qualitative information about a program. When used together for the same purpose, the quantitative and qualitative methods build on each other and offer insights that neither one alone can offer (King et al. 1994; Mark and Shotland 1987; Reichardt and Cook 1979; Shortell 1999). Put another way, all research methods have their own biases, and using quantitative and qualitative methods in tandem helps to correct for the biases and shortcomings in each one. Because the methods are so different, the evaluator also is in a better position to triangulate their findings and arrive at the "underlying truth" (Reichardt and Cook 1979).

For example, using a regression discontinuity impact design (see Chapter 4), a community-based intervention is planned to raise public awareness and reduce the sale of illegal drugs on the street corners of a city neighborhood (Reichardt and Cook 1979). The neighborhood is defined by a boundary; households inside the boundary receive the intervention, and households outside the boundary do not. To determine whether the intervention is working, ethnographers wander back and forth across the boundary to determine if there was a discontinuity in awareness or purchase of illegal drugs.

Qualitative methods also can yield insights about the best ways to construct a quantitative measure of a concept. For example, Grembowski et al. (1993) developed questionnaire items for measuring the self-efficacy of older adults in performing health-promoting behaviors. Collected mainly from English-speaking, Caucasian patients in private medical clinics, the items might not be culturally suitable for patients with diverse ethnic or racial backgrounds in other health care settings. Focused interviews or other qualitative methods could be used to collect information about the questionnaire items and about what "self-efficacy" means to these individuals. This information could then be used to revise the items, which could then be tested for reliability and validity as described earlier in this chapter.

Alternatively, an evaluator may choose to construct an "unobtrusive" quantitative measure about the outcomes of a health program through the collection of qualitative information (Webb et al. 1966). For example, suppose a company launches a health promotion program to reduce cigarette smoking among its employees. To evaluate the program's impact, employees will be asked about their smoking behavior in a follow-up questionnaire. The evaluators are concerned that some smokers, who want to please their employer, may report smoking fewer cigarettes when, in fact, their smoking has stayed the same or increased. The evaluators therefore use qualitative methods to monitor the use of ashtrays, which becomes a second, unobtrusive measure of program outcomes.

Although using both quantitative and qualitative methods is desirable, several barriers may block their usage in health program evaluation (Reichardt and Cook 1979). Using both methods increases the costs and time to complete an evaluation relative to using either one alone. Furthermore, the evaluator must be versed in both methods, or personnel with the missing expertise must be added to the evaluation team. Although these barriers can loom large in many evaluations, they can be surmounted by focusing quantitative-qualitative data collection on a few critical questions, such as impact results that will likely show small differences at best between the intervention and control group, or a question that, when answered, will likely generate much political controversy in Act III of the evaluation process.

Reliability and Validity in Qualitative Evaluations

Although reliability and validity assessments of quantitative measures are performed before data collection begins, these assessments in qualitative evaluations are performed either before, during, or after data collection is under way. Different methods exist for assessing the reliability and validity of qualitative measures (Caudle 1994; Kirk 1986; Maxwell 1998; Silverman et al. 1990). Focusing on reliability assessments, one aim is to determine whether information collected at different points in time is the same or different. Thus, the reliability of qualitative information collected from key informants can be verified by re-interviewing the informant and verifying whether responses are consistent. Formal field debriefing, where evaluation staff discuss the information collected to verify interpretations and identify themes, is another method for assessing the reliability of the interpretations of the data. Evidence of reliability exists if different people examine the same information and identify the same themes. Methods for assessing the reliability of observers were described earlier in this chapter.

Similarly, a variety of methods exist for assessing the validity of qualitative information. Common methods, which typically entail some form of triangulation, are described below. In most triangulation methods, evidence of validity exists when the results are congruent and/or complement each other (Caudle 1994). Congruence occurs when different evidence yields similar, consistent results. Complementarity exists when one set of results expands on or clarifies the results from another source of information.

▶ *Multiple discipline triangulation* is one method that takes different forms. If the evaluation team is composed of investigators from multiple disciplines, the qualitative information is critically reviewed and interpreted from more than one perspective to reveal any biases inherent in any single perspective. Similarly, the validity of information collected from key informants can be assessed by interviewing a person over several sessions, each time with a different interviewer from a different discipline. For example, the nurse practitioner that runs a high school clinic could receive an in-depth interview from an evaluator with a social science background and a second interview by an evaluator with a clinical background.

▶ *Methods triangulation* entails finding similar results from different methods, which may include different data sources, data collection procedures, different measures, and different qualitative methods. This form of triangulation includes comparing qualitative results with the evaluation's quantitative results for consistency. An example of methods triangulation, a community-based intervention about illegal drug sales, was presented earlier.

▶ *Theory triangulation* occurs when initial results are congruent with an existing theory. For example, focused interviews with uninsured adults may indicate they have tremendous difficulty finding medical care for their health problems, which is consistent with economic theory.

▶ *Rival explanations* entail the systematic search for rival or competing themes or explanations that do not conform with initial interpretations of the data. One form of this approach is negative case analysis (Caudle 1994). For example, a new health education curriculum in 20 high schools might reveal initially that students learn more when teachers closely follow the curriculum. To verify the trustworthiness of this finding, classes are identified where the teacher did not follow the curriculum but students still had significant knowledge gains. These classes are examined intensively to understand why they do not conform to the overall results.

▶ *Evidence weighting* means giving more weight to stronger data and discarding or downplaying evidence that is weak. Examples of stronger data include data that come from the most knowledgeable informants, that are based on behavior seen or reported at first hand, or that a respondent volunteers when alone with the evaluator.

▶ *Field debriefing*, as described earlier, may lead to the identification of conflicting interpretations or biases among those collecting the data in the field.

▶ *Feedback* to an advisory board or another peer group is another method for verifying whether the data are accurate and whether interpretations are consistent with the evidence.

In summary, different methods exist for assessing the reliability and validity of qualitative data. These methods can be applied individually or in combination to improve the trustworthiness of the evaluation.

MANAGEMENT OF DATA COLLECTION

Once data collection is under way, the management of data collection activities becomes the focus of the evaluation. Sound management of data collection requires knowledge and experience in planning and budgeting; hiring and training qualified staff to collect the data; supervising staff; installing quality control checks to ensure the integrity of data collection; developing and managing paper and information flows; coding, editing, and entering data into computer files; designing and managing the evaluation's database; and documenting all the data collection protocols and data files that result from the evaluation (Bell 1994; Bourque and Clark 1992; St. Pierre 1983; Stouthamer-Loeber and van Kammen 1995). In general, as the scope of the evaluation increases, so does the importance of proper management of data collection, particularly if the evaluation *must* be completed by a specific date and within a fixed budget. The ultimate goal of data collection is to produce the database that will be analyzed to answer the questions of the evaluation. Thus, although data collection and database construction may lack the glamour and excitement of designing the evaluation itself, the evaluation cannot be completed without this essential step.

SUMMARY

Once the target populations and samples are selected, the next step in the evaluation process is to identify and collect information about each one to answer all the evaluation questions about the program. Information about health programs can be collected through quantitative or qualitative methods, and evaluations are more rigorous when both methods are used in tandem. In quantitative evaluations, the ultimate goal of measurement and data collection is to produce a database that contains a limited amount of information for a large number of people, which the evaluator uses to answer the questions about the program. To build the database, the evaluator must decide what concepts to measure, identify measures of those concepts, assess the quality of the measures, identify the data source of each measure, make final decisions about what measures to keep and reject, and finally collect the measures. Completing these steps requires sound conceptual, methodological, and management skills; attention to details; and a clear picture of what the evaluation's database will look like in the end.

In contrast, qualitative evaluations typically produce rich, detailed information about the program from a much smaller number of people. Qualitative information can be used to understand the experiences of people in the program, to define and construct quantitative measures, to obtain unobtrusive measures about the program, or to complement the findings from an impact evaluation. The reliability and validity of qualitative information can be assessed through different methods to improve the trustworthiness of the evaluation.

Once data collection is completed, data analyses are ready to begin. These are addressed in the next chapter.

RESOURCES

Qualitative Research References

Bryman A, Burgess R. *Qualitative Research* (Vols. I-IV). Thousand Oaks, CA: Sage; 1999.

Creswell JW. *Qualitative Inquiry and Research Design: Choosing Among Five Traditions.* Thousand Oaks, CA: Sage; 1997.

Denzin NK, Lincoln YS. *Handbook of Qualitative Research.* Thousand Oaks, CA: Sage; 2000.

Grbich C. *Qualitative Research in Health: An Introduction.* Thousand Oaks, CA: Sage; 1998.

King G, Keohane RO, Verba S. *Designing Social Inquiry: Scientific Inference in Qualitative Research*. Princeton, NJ: Princeton University Press; 1994.

Krueger RA, Casey MA. *Focus Groups: A Practical Guide for Applied Research*. Thousand Oaks, CA: Sage; 2000.

Lofland J, Lofland LH. *Analyzing Social Settings: A Guide to Qualitative Observation and Analysis*. Belmont, CA: Wadsworth Publishing; 1984.

Miles MB, Huberman M. *Qualitative Data Analysis: An Expanded Sourcebook*. Thousand Oaks, CA: Sage; 1994.

Morgan DL. *Successful Focus Groups: Advancing the State of the Art*. Thousand Oaks, CA: Sage; 1993.

Morse JM, Field PA. *Qualitative Research Methods for Health Professionals*. Thousand Oaks, CA: Sage; 1995.

Patton MQ. *How to Use Qualitative Methods in Evaluation*. Thousand Oaks, CA: Sage; 1987.

Seale C. *The Quality of Qualitative Research*. Thousand Oaks, CA: Sage; 1999.

Stewart A. *The Ethnographer's Method*. Thousand Oaks, CA: Sage; 1998.

Health Services References

Aday LA, Andersen R. *Development of Indices of Access to Medical Care*. Ann Arbor, MI: Health Administration Press; 1975.

Andersen RM, Davidson PL. Measuring access and trends. In: Anderson RM, Rice TH, Kominski GF, eds. *Changing the U.S. Health Care System: Key Issues in Health Services, Policy and Management*. San Francisco: Jossey-Bass; 1996:13-40.

Brown JB, Adams ME. Patients as reliable reporters of medical care process: Recall of ambulatory encounter events. *Medical Care* 1992; 30(5):400-411.

Center for Health Economics Research. *Access to Health Care: Key Indicators for Policy*. Princeton, NJ: Robert Wood Johnson Foundation; 1993.

DeFriese GH, Ricketts TC, Stein JS. *Methodological Advances in Health Services Research*. Ann Arbor, MI: Health Administration Press; 1989.

Farrow DC, Connell FA. A comparison of measures of prenatal care use. *Medical Care* 1997; 35(3):297-300.

Miller DC. *Handbook of Research Design and Social Measurement*. Thousand Oaks, CA: Sage; 1991.

Nunnally JC, Bernstein IH. *Psychometric Theory*. New York: McGraw-Hill; 1994.

Rice TH. Measuring health care costs and trends. In Anderson RM, Rice TH, Kominski GF, eds. *Changing the U.S. Health Care System: Key Issues in*

Health Services, Policy and Management. San Francisco: Jossey-Bass; 1996:62-80.

Stouthamer-Loeber M, Van Kammen WB. *Data Collection and Management: A Practical Guide.* Thousand Oaks, CA: Sage; 1995.

Wallihan DB. Accuracy of self-reported health services use and patterns of care among urban older adults. *Medical Care* 1999; 37(7):662-670.

Survey References

Aday LA. *Designing and Conducting Health Surveys.* San Francisco: Jossey-Bass; 1996.

Bourque LB, Clark VA. *Processing Data: The Survey Example.* Newbury Park, CA: Sage; 1992.

Converse JM, Presser S. *Survey Questions: Handcrafting the Standardized Questionnaire.* Newbury Park, CA: Sage; 1986.

Dillman DA. *Mail and Telephone Surveys: The Total Design Method.* New York: John Wiley; 1978.

Dillman DA. *Mail and Electronic Surveys: The Tailored Design Method.* New York: John Wiley and Sons; 1999.

Fink A, Kosecoff J. *How to Conduct Surveys: A Step-by-Step Guide.* Newbury Park, CA: Sage; 1985.

Fowler FJ. *Survey Research Methods.* 2nd ed. Newbury Park, CA: Sage; 1988, 1993.

Fowler FJ, Mangione TW. *Standardized Survey Interviewing: Minimizing Interviewer-Related Error.* Newbury Park, CA: Sage; 1989.

Frey JH. *Survey Research by Telephone.* Newbury Park, CA: Sage; 1983.

Lavrakas PJ. *Telephone Survey Methods: Sampling, Selection, and Supervision.* Newbury Park, CA: Sage; 1993.

Mavis BE, Bocato JJ. Postal surveys versus electronic mail surveys: The tortoise and the hare revisited. *Evaluation and the Health Professions* 1998; 21(3):395-408.

Rosenfeld JE, Thomas MD, Thomas E. *Improving Organizational Surveys.* Newbury Park, CA: Sage; 1993.

Salant P, Dillman DA. *How to Conduct Your Own Survey.* New York: John Wiley and Sons; 1994.

Schaefer DR, Dillman DA. Development of a standard e-mail methodology: Results of an experiment. *Public Opinion Quarterly* 1998; 62:378-397.

Sudman S, Bradburn NM. *Asking Questions: A Practical Guide to Questionnaire Design.* San Francisco: Jossey-Bass; 1982.

Measurement of Health Status

Bowling A. *Measuring Disease: A Review of Disease-Specific Quality of Life Measurement Scales.* Philadelphia: Open University Press; 1995.

Ganz PA, Litwin MS. Measuring outcomes and health-related quality of life. In: Anderson RM, Rice TH, Kominski GF, eds. *Changing the U.S. Health Care System: Key Issues in Health Services, Policy and Management.* San Francisco: Jossey-Bass; 1996:120-141.

Kane RL. *Understanding Health Care Outcomes Research.* Gaithersburg, MD: Aspen; 1997.

Larson JS. *The Measurement of Health: Concepts and Indicators.* New York: Greenwood Press; 1991.

Lohr KN. Outcome measurement: Concepts and questions. *Inquiry* 1988; 25(Spring):37-50.

Lorig K, Stewart A, Ritter P, Gonzalez V, Laurent D, Lynch J. *Outcome Measures for Health Education and Other Health Care Interventions.* Thousand Oaks, CA: Sage; 1996.

Patrick DL, Erickson P. *Health Status and Health Policy: Quality of Life in Health Care Evaluation and Resource Allocation.* New York: Oxford University Press; 1993.

Stewart AL, Ware JE Jr. *Measuring Functioning and Well-Being: The Medical Outcomes Study Approach.* Durham, NC: Duke University Press; 1992.

Streiner DL, Norman GR. *Health Measurement Scales: A Practical Guide to Their Development and Use.* New York: Oxford University Press; 1995.

Wilkin D, Hallam L, Doggett M. *Measures of Need and Outcome for Primary Health Care.* New York: Oxford University Press; 1992.

Measurement of Patient Satisfaction

Chapko M, et al. Development and validation of a measure of dental patient satisfaction. *Medical Care* 1985; 23:39-49.

Corah NL, O'Shea RM, Pace LF, Seyrek SK. Development of a patient measure of satisfaction with the dentist: The dental visit satisfaction scale. *Journal of Behavioral Medicine* 1984; 7:367-373.

Davies AR, Ware JE Jr. *Development of a Dental Satisfaction Questionnaire for the Health Insurance Experiment.* Publication No. R-2712-HHS. Santa Monica, CA: Rand Corporation; 1982.

Hayes R, Baker DW. Methodological problems in comparing English-speaking and Spanish-speaking patients' satisfaction with interpersonal aspects of care. *Medical Care* 1998; 36(2):230-236.

Loeken K, Steine S, Sandvik L, Laerum E. A new instrument to measure patient satisfaction with mammography: Validity, reliability, and discriminatory power. *Medical Care* 1997; 35(7):731-741.

Patrick DL, Erickson P. *Health Status and Health Policy: Quality of Life in Health Care Evaluation and Resource Allocation.* New York: Oxford University Press; 1993.

Roberts JG, Tugwell P. Comparison of questionnaires determining patient satisfaction with medical care. *Health Services Research* 1987; 637-654.

Ross CK, Steward CA, Sinacore JM. A comparative study of seven measures of patient satisfaction. *Medical Care* 1995; 33(4):392-406.

Rubin HR, Gandek B, Rogers WH, Kosinski M, McHorney CA, Ware JE Jr. Patients' ratings of outpatient visits in different practice settings. *JAMA* 1993; 270(7):835-840.

Sisk JE, Gorman SA, Reisinger AL, Glied SA, DuMouchel WH, Hynes MM. Evaluation of Medicaid managed care: Satisfaction, access and use. *JAMA* 1996; 276(1):50-55.

Steiber SR, Krowinski WJ. *Measuring and Managing Patient Satisfaction.* Chicago: American Hospital Association; 1990.

Strasser S, Davis RM. *Measuring Patient Satisfaction for Improved Patient Services.* Ann Arbor, MI: Health Administration Press; 1991.

Van Campen C, Sixma H, Friele RD, Kerssens JJ, Peters L. Quality of care and patient satisfaction: A review of measuring instruments. *Medical Care Research and Review* 1995; 52(1):109-133.

Ware JE Jr., Hays RD. Methods for measuring patient satisfaction with specific medical encounters. *Medical Care* 1988; 26(4):393-402.

Ware JE Jr., Snyder MK, Wright R, Davies AR. Defining and measuring patient satisfaction with medical care. *Evaluation and Program Planning* 1983; 6:247-263.

Measurement of Health Behavior

Donovan DM, Marlatt GA. *Assessment of Addictive Behaviors.* New York: Guilford Press; 1988.

Glanz K, Lewis FM, Rimer BK. *Health Education and Health Behavior: Theory, Research, and Practice.* San Francisco: Jossey-Bass; 1996.

Karoly P. *Measurement Strategies in Health Psychology.* New York: Wiley; 1985.

Lorig K, Stewart A, Ritter P, Gonzalez V, Laurent D, Lynch J. *Outcome Measures for Health Education and Other Health Care Interventions.* Thousand Oaks, CA: Sage; 1996.

Robinson J, Shaver P, Wrightsman L. *Measures of Personality and Social Psychological Attitudes* (Vol. I). San Diego: Academic Press; 1991.

LIST OF TERMS _____

Alternative-form reliability	Measurement levels
Classification	Multiple disciplines
Concept	Nominal measurement level
Constant	Nonrandom error
Construct validity	Operational definition
Content validity	Ordinal measurement level
Criterion validity	Primary data source
Data sources	Program variable
Debriefing	Qualitative validity assessment
Dependent variable	Random error
Evidence weighting	Ratio measurement level
Face validity	Reliability
Feedback	Reliability coefficient
Independent control variable	Responsiveness
Internal consistency	Rival explanations
Interrater/interobserver reliability	Secondary data source
Interval measurement level	Split-half reliability
Intrarater/intraobserver reliability	Test-retest reliability
Measure	Triangulation
Measurement	Validity
Measurement error	Variable

1. What are measurement reliability and validity? How are they related to internal validity?

2. Can a measure be unreliable but still be valid?

3. How do a program's measures affect the data collection and data analysis plan?

4. Why is variation important in choosing a measure?

5. When would you employ only qualitative methods to answer an evaluation question vs. using both quantitative and qualitative methods?

6. What are two ways that triangulation can be used to verify the validity of findings in a qualitative evaluation?

CHAPTER 9

Data Analysis

At this point in Act II of the evaluation process, major milestones have been achieved. By now the evaluation team has a clear understanding of the health program and its goals and objectives. Key questions about the program have been posed, and one or more evaluation designs exist for answering each question. The target populations for each question have been identified, and the sampling protocols for each population have been carried out. Qualitative data collection is under way. The evaluation team has identified quantitative measures with known reliability, validity, and responsiveness that they want to collect from each population or sample. Data collection protocols have been implemented to collect the measures, and a database exists that contains the information to answer each question. The next and final step in Act II of the evaluation process is to analyze the data to produce results, or new information, that answers each question. In many evaluations, this is an exciting time filled with discovery as new insights about the program emerge. It also can be a very satisfying time for the evaluation team as the hard work of collecting and analyzing the data yields the final conclusions, or "bottom line," of the evaluation.

The purpose of this chapter is to examine key issues in organizing and conducting analyses of qualitative and quantitative data collected in health program evaluations. The chapter begins with a "question-oriented" strategy for organizing data analysis. Next, qualitative data analysis and its role in health program evaluation are reviewed. Finally, issues in quantitative data analysis are reviewed. The specific techniques for analyzing qualitative and quantitative data are beyond the scope of this textbook, and students are advised to complete separate courses devoted to those topics.

GETTING STARTED: WHAT'S THE QUESTION?

In the data collection phase of the evaluation, the attention of the evaluation team is focused intensively on the details of collecting information and building a database. This work often produces a "mountain" of information about the program that can take myriad forms—minutes from program staff meetings, interviews of program clients, information from focus groups, medical claims from public and private insurance agencies, information abstracted from patient charts, responses to surveys, and so on—depending on the program. Buried with data, the evaluation team faces a real danger of "losing sight of the forest," or becoming lost in the data with no clear direction about what to do with all the information that has been collected (Shortell and Richardson 1978). At one extreme, the evaluation team may be overwhelmed with the data and "freeze up," and few analyses are performed. At the other extreme, the evaluation team may examine all possible combinations of all possible variables, which only creates even more information and confusion that prevent the team from making sense of the data that were collected originally. In general, most databases have a story to tell, and evaluation teams must find a strategy for analyzing the data that reveals the story embedded within it.

One strategy that works for many health programs is to develop a "question-oriented" data analysis plan. In Act I of the evaluation process, decision makers asked specific questions about the program, and the aim of the data analysis is to produce the information that answers each one. To fulfill this aim, the data analysis must be "question-oriented"—that is, organized to identify the information in the database that is required to answer a question, analyze this information using one or more appropriate techniques, and formulate an answer to the question based on the results. This strategy also provides a structure for packaging and disseminating answers to decision makers in Act III of the evaluation process, addressed in the next chapter.

Fleming and Andersen (1986) provide an excellent example of "question-oriented" data analysis in their evaluation of the Municipal Health Services Program (MHSP), a demonstration program funded by the Robert Wood Johnson Foundation to determine whether installing primary care clinics in inner-city locations would improve access to primary care for the low-income people who live there without increasing expenditures. The evaluation was designed to answer the following questions about the demonstration:

▶ Did the MHSP reach the groups it was intended to serve?

▶ Did the MHSP increase access for patients?

▶ Was care appropriate?

▶ Were patients satisfied?

▶ Did MHSP reduce expenditures?

In the results section of their article, Fleming and Andersen highlight the first question of the evaluation and then present the evidence that answers it. Then, the second question is posed, and the evidence that answers the question is presented. This cycle is repeated until all the questions are answered. After all the results are known, the answers to all the questions become the information base for judging the overall merits of the demonstration.

QUALITATIVE DATA ANALYSIS

In qualitative evaluations of health programs, the main goals often are to understand what has happened in the program and why, and to understand the program from the participant's perspective (Patton 1987; Weiss 1998a). The chief method of accomplishing these goals is inductive inquiry, trying to identify major themes in the vast amounts of field data, which may be in the form of observation records, interview responses, focus group transcripts, tapes, abstracts of documents, or other field notes (Caudle 1994; Weiss 1998a). In qualitative methods, data collection and data analysis are not separate activities (Weiss 1998a). In the field, data analysis begins as data are collected. Emerging themes and insights are noted, partly to gain an understanding of the program and partly because what is learned early about the program can influence what is collected from whom later in the data collection process. When data collection is completed in the field, a number of analytical techniques can be used to examine the data; these are described in detail in the qualitative methods literature (see references at the end of Chapter 8). Computer software also is available for analyzing qualitative data in ways that can be reproduced by others (Caudle 1994).

To answer an evaluation question, all the qualitative information for answering the question should be identified by reviewing the evaluation's conceptual model and the information requirements of the implementation evaluation design. Next, evaluators should acquire a firsthand knowledge of the contents of the qualitative information that will be used to answer each question. Because qualitative information is often text rather than numbers, this can be more time-consuming, difficult, and painstaking work than the analysis of quantitative variables. If text information is analyzed and coded in numeric form, the distributions of these variables and their associations also should be examined.

When the final inferences begin to form, the evaluator uses triangulation to cross-check their accuracy. As introduced in Chapter 8, Denzin (1978) describes four types of triangulation that can be used either individually or in combination with each other:

1. Data triangulation asks the question "Do different sources of data yield similar results?" For example, do interviews of program managers vs. staff yield similar findings?
2. Investigator triangulation asks the question "If the data are examined by different evaluators or social scientists from different disciplines (such as a sociologist, an economist, and a psychologist), are the findings and conclusions similar across investigators?"
3. Theory triangulation asks the question "If different theories are used to interpret a set of data, are the results similar or different?"
4. Methodological triangulation asks the question "If different methods—such as interviews, observations, questionnaires, and document reviews—are used to evaluate a health program, is the evidence across the methods consistent or conflicting?"

Evaluators generally have more confidence in the accuracy of their findings when triangulation yields consistent findings and conclusions across different data sources, methods, theories, or investigators (Patton 1987).

Qualitative analyses produce results that can assume myriad forms that are inherently descriptive (Caudle 1994; Miles and Huberman 1984, 1994; Patton 1987). Qualitative analysis can be performed to portray the "culture" of the program, to compare different parts of the program, to find commonalities among the parts, to examine deviant cases, to rule out rival explanations for patterns found in quantitative analyses, or simply "to tell the story" of what has gone on in the program (Weiss 1998a). If the qualitative data are coded in numeric form, they also can be included in the quantitative analyses described in the next section.

More specifically, the findings from qualitative analyses can be used to answer three basic types of evaluation questions (also see Chapter 6). First, qualitative findings can be the sole source, or just one of multiple sources, of information to answer a question about a program's implementation. For example, in the evaluation of the high school clinic, the student focus groups could be the only source of information to answer an evaluation question about whether students are satisfied with the clinic, or the focus group information could be combined with satisfaction information collected through a student survey to answer the evaluation question.

Second, qualitative findings can be used to explain the outcomes obtained in an impact evaluation. For example, to reduce unintended teen pregnancy and reduce sexually transmitted diseases, 10 Seattle high schools made condoms available through vending machines or baskets in their high school clinics (Kirby et al. 1999). The implementation results showed that 133,711 condoms were distributed, or an average of 4.6 condoms per student during the school year. The impact results showed, however, that the distribution of condoms did not increase sexual activity, nor did it increase condom use. To explain these contradictory results, 16 focus groups from the high schools were conducted, and the following themes emerged (Brown et al. 1997):

▶ A key assumption of the intervention (that is, a part of its theory of cause and effect) was that condoms were not available to students, and increasing availability might result in greater use of condoms and reduced pregnancies and sexually transmitted diseases. The focus groups revealed, however, that condoms were already available to students before the schools began offering them. Hence, a "substitution effect" occurred, with the high schools replacing the students' previous sources of condoms.

▶ The intervention did not address the reasons why students do not use condoms (such as "didn't plan ahead," "trusted partner," and so forth).

▶ The students themselves did not think the program affected their sexual activity or condom use.

Similarly, in the Medicare demonstration described in Chapter 6, qualitative evidence from medical charts was used to understand why Medicare enrollees in the intervention group had a higher mortality rate than the control group.

Third, qualitative findings also are useful for confirming or disproving a program's theory of cause and effect or theory of implementation (Weiss 1998a). In the lead poisoning program described in Chapter 3, for example, the program's "chain of events" posited that the repair of housing in low-income neighborhoods would reduce children's exposure to lead, which usually occurred when young children ate chips of lead-based paint that peeled from tenement walls. Although the incidence of lead poisoning decreased following the program, the decline was not due to the house repairs. Instead, qualitative information revealed that, as a result of the publicity about the program, parents monitored their children's behavior more closely, taking paint chips away when their children picked them up.

QUANTITATIVE DATA ANALYSIS

What Are the Variables for Answering Each Question?

Quantitative data analysis begins with identifying all the quantitative information, or variables, that the evaluator plans to use for answering each question. This can be done by revisiting the evaluation's conceptual model and impact and implementation designs, reviewing their concepts and the variables that measure them, and making preliminary decisions about what variables to include and exclude in the data analysis for each question.

Next, it is imperative for the evaluator to "get close to the data" and develop a firsthand knowledge of the distribution of each variable that is used to answer each question (Shortell and Richardson 1978). Analysis of distributions means computing and inspecting basic descriptive statistics, such as the mean, standard deviation, range, and kurtosis (a measure of skewness in the distribution), as well as constructing and examining histograms of each variable. This knowledge is vital to choosing the proper statistical technique for analyzing the data. For example, let's suppose that total annual medical expenditures is a key dependent variable for the evaluation of a health program. Inspection of the variable's histogram reveals that 30% of the individuals had zero expenditures for medical care in the past year, while the expenditures for the remaining 70% have a skewed distribution. This information is important because parametric statistical techniques usually assume that the dependent variable has a normal distribution. When this is not the case, other analytical techniques must be considered. For example, annual medical expenditures could be recoded to create a new, binary (0, 1) variable, where "0" indicates that an individual had no medical expenditures in the past year and "1" indicates that the individual had expenditures. Data analyses could then be conducted with statistical methods, such as chi-square or logistic regression, that are appropriate for binary dependent measures.

In addition, analysis of distributions is also useful for detecting data entry or coding errors that may still exist in the database. For example, if the distribution for annual medical expenditures reveals that three individuals had much higher expenditures than others, the medical claims for those individuals should be inspected to determine whether a coding error occurred, or whether the data were entered incorrectly.

Based on the analysis of the distributions, some variables may be recoded to create new variables, and other variables that exhibit little variation may be dropped from the analysis. Once all the variables for answering a question are specified, they should be categorized as either dependent, program, or control variables (see Chapter 8). Furthermore, each dependent variable should be classified by its level of measurement—nominal, interval (or categorical), ordinal, or ratio (see Chapter 8). This classification is important because the choice of statistical techniques for answering a question depends partly on the dependent variable's level of measurement.

Personal computer software from a variety of companies can be purchased to perform quantitative analyses. With the advent of advanced and yet easy-to-use software packages, there is a temptation to proceed directly to the higher-level procedures to obtain the "final answer" for an evaluation question. The problem with this approach, however, is that proper use of the advanced procedures normally requires a thorough understanding of the details of the variables in the database. Furthermore, if this knowledge is not developed at an early stage, there is no foundation for making informed decisions about how to perform the advanced procedures and how to interpret the results obtained from them. In short, putting in the time and work to become well acquainted with the database early on yields dividends downstream when the analyses for answering each question are performed.

How Should the Variables Be Analyzed?

In general, there are three types of quantitative data analysis: *descriptive*, *bivariable*, and *multivariable*. One or all three types of data analysis may be performed to answer an evaluation question. Choosing the type of data analysis depends on several factors; some key concerns include the following:

▶ *Who is the audience?* If the primary audience for the evaluation results is composed of program officials, program clients, advisory groups, and local decision makers, simple descriptive or bivariable analyses are often sufficient. If, however, the results are directed at outside evaluation experts, a funding agency, or a journal for publication, more rigorous multivariable analyses may be warranted.

▶ *How political is the evaluation?* If political controversy surrounds an evaluation and the evaluation findings do not support the positions of one or more interest groups, the evaluation findings may be attacked by the groups in the next act of the evaluation process. If controversy is likely no matter what the evaluation findings are, more rigorous methods of data analysis are warranted.

▶ *Does the impact evaluation have a randomized design?* If an impact evaluation uses a randomized design to create balanced treatment and control groups, bivariable analyses may be sufficient to determine whether a significant difference exists in the outcomes between the two groups. On the other hand, if an impact evaluation uses a nonrandomized design, multivariable analyses are warranted to control for other factors that might also account for program outcomes.

▶ *What type of analysis is appropriate to answer the question?* If an evaluator has an in-depth knowledge of regression analysis, the evaluator may automatically use this technique to answer a question because it is what the evaluator knows best. To avoid this tendency, which is known as the "law of the instrument" (Kaplan 1964), evaluators should be well versed in a variety of analytical techniques and selectively choose techniques based on their ability to produce the evidence required to answer a given question.

Descriptive analysis includes the quantitative analysis of distributions described earlier, as well as most forms of qualitative data analysis. As its name implies, the aim of descriptive analysis is simply to describe the data that answer a question. The following hypothetical questions about a clinic located in a high school may be answered by conducting descriptive analyses of the data collected in the evaluation. In descriptive designs for implementation evaluation (see Chapter 6), descriptive analysis may be all that is necessary to answer these kinds of basic questions about health programs.

Question	Descriptive Analysis
What percentage of students visited the high school clinic at least once?	Frequency distribution of clinic visits
Are students who visited the clinic satisfied with the services they received?	Average clinic satisfaction score
Why are some students dissatisfied with the clinic?	Major themes identified from focus groups composed of dissatisfied students

Bivariable analysis is performed to determine whether two variables are associated with each other. Two basic types of bivariable analyses typically are performed in health program evaluations. The aim of the first type of bivariable analysis is to determine whether variables in the database are correlated with each other. The statistical test for calculating the correlation depends on the level of measurement of the two variables. Pearson correlation may be used for two interval or ratio variables, such as years of education and annual income. Spearman correlation, Kendall's tau, and gamma can be used to determine whether two ordinal variables are associated with each other, such as self-rated health and rating of health care (both measured on an ordinal scale such as excellent, very good, good, fair, or poor). A chi-square test can be performed to determine whether two nominal variables, such as gender and race, are associated with each other.

The second type of bivariable analysis is performed when we want to *compare* two or more groups to find out whether a characteristic is similar or different across the groups. This type of bivariable analysis is performed frequently in explanatory designs of implementation evaluation (see Chapter 6). For example, in the evaluation of the high school clinic, the question may be asked, "Who uses the clinic more, freshmen or seniors?" In this example, the two groups are the freshman and the senior classes, and we want to compare clinic use between the two classes over the past school year. One way to compare the two classes is to perform a *t* test to find out whether the average number of clinic visits among students in the freshmen class is significantly different from the average number of clinic visits among students in the senior class. Alternatively, a chi-square test could be performed comparing the percentage of freshmen who visited the clinic at least once in the past year with the percentage of seniors who visited the clinic at least once. Given nominal variables, the chi-square test also can be used to determine whether the percentage of students visiting the clinic is significantly different among all four classes (freshmen, sophomores, juniors, and seniors). If the characteristic is an interval or ratio variable, however, such as the number of visits in the school year, and two or more classes are compared, analysis of variance can be used to determine whether the average number of visits is significantly different across the classes.

The second type of bivariable analysis also can be conducted in impact evaluations to find out *whether* program outcomes are significantly different between groups or within one group over time. Depending on the impact design, three types of comparisons of program outcomes can be performed (Dennis 1994):

▶ *A comparison of baseline and outcome scores for members of the treatment group, such as in the pretest-posttest design.* For example, if interval or ratio variables are used to measure outcomes, and if a person's pretest observation can be linked with the person's posttest observation in the database, a paired *t* test can be performed to determine whether a significant difference exists between the pretest and posttest scores of the individuals.

▶ *A comparison of outcomes in the treatment group with the outcomes of the comparison group at a single point in time, such as in the posttest-only comparison group design or the posttest-only control group design.* For example, in a posttest-only control group design with outcomes measured at the ratio level, a *t* test can be performed to determine whether the average outcome in the treatment group is significantly different from the average outcome in the comparison group. The bivariable statistical test is appropriate if we assume that randomization in fact created equivalent groups and thereby eliminated the need to control statistically for other factors that might influence program outcomes.

▶ *A comparison of the change in outcomes in the treatment group with the change in outcomes in another group, such as in the pretest-posttest control group design or the nonequivalent comparison group design.* For example, in the Medicare demonstration, which used a pretest-posttest control group design, the average change between the pretest and posttest scores for adults in the treatment group can be computed, along with the average change between the scores for the adults in the control group. Then, a *t* test can be performed to determine whether a statistically significant difference exists between the average change scores of the two groups. Results revealed that at the 24-month and 48-month follow-ups, the intervention group exercised more, consumed less dietary fat, and completed more advanced directives. As reported earlier, more deaths occurred in the intervention group. Surviving treatment-group members reported higher satisfaction with health, less decline in self-rated health status, and fewer depressive symptoms than surviving control-group members. The intervention did not lower health care costs (Patrick et al. 1999).

One shortcoming of bivariable statistical tests is that they indicate only *whether or not* two variables are significantly different from each other. Thus, if the outcome of the treatment group is significantly different from the outcome of the control group, bivariable analyses cannot estimate the *size* of the program's effect on observed outcomes. Another shortcoming of bivariable tests is that they do not control for other factors besides the program that also may account for observed outcomes. This is a critical disadvantage for nonrandomized impact designs where selection is a threat to internal validity.

To overcome these drawbacks, multivariable analysis can be performed to estimate the size and direction of a program's effect in impact designs with a treatment and control group. Multivariable analyses typically employ regression models to estimate program effects, where the type of regression model depends on the level of measurement of the dependent variable. In a posttest-only comparison group design, the general form of the regression model for estimating program effects is

$$O = f(T, C, I) \tag{9.1}$$

where
O = Outcome variable
T = (0, 1) is a dummy variable
where 1 = member of treatment group
and 0 = member of the comparison group
C = Control variables
I = One or more interaction terms

If the regression coefficient for the T ("treatment group") variable is statistically significant, the T coefficient is the estimate of the program's effect. The value of the coefficient indicates the size of the effect, and the sign of the coefficient, positive or negative, indicates the direction of the effect. For example, let's assume the outcome variable is "patient satisfaction with the program," which is measured on a 0-to-10 scale, where "10" is highly satisfied. Let's also assume the T coefficient equals 0.50 and is positive. This finding indicates that, on average, individuals in the treatment group were about a half a point more satisfied on the 0-to-10 point satisfaction scale than individuals in the comparison group, controlling for the variables in the C-vector.

The regression model also includes interaction terms to determine whether program effects vary across subgroups (Jaccard et al. 1990; Shortell and Richardson 1978). For example, if the program has a statistically significant effect, a question may be raised about whether the effect is the same or different for men and women. To answer this question, an interaction variable, the multiplication of T and the binary (0, 1) gender variable, is included in the model to test statistically for the presence or absence of this interaction effect.

Selection is a key threat to internal validity in the posttest-only comparison group design (see Chapter 4) and may produce biased estimates of program effects (the T coefficient in Equation 9.1). This is because, under self-selection, individuals who may have a comparative advantage with the program may be more likely to join the program and thus may benefit more from it than randomly selected persons with the same characteristics (Maddala 1983). To address this problem, evaluators may apply statistical techniques developed mainly in economics to correct for potential selection bias (Maddala 1983). One statistical approach is to employ "switching regression models," which usually entail the estimation of two regression equations (Berk 1983). The first equation is a "choice equation" containing independent variables that explain participation or nonparticipation in the program. The parameter estimates from the choice equation are then used to predict each person's probability of not participating in the program, a variable known as the "hazard rate." The hazard rate is then inserted as an additional variable into Equation 9.1 to correct for potential self-selection.

A second approach to correct for selection bias is known as "instrumental variables" (Newhouse and McClellan 1998). The basic idea is to define a variable, or "instrument," that accounts for a person's selection into the program *but has no direct effect on program outcomes*. For example, suppose an HMO develops a special clinic for treating all members of its population with diabetes, and the HMO wants to find out if patients who attend the clinic have better health outcomes than those who do not. Suppose also that the distance between a diabetic's residence and the clinic is a key determinant of whether a patient visits the clinic, and that distance is unrelated to health outcomes. In this case, distance is an instrument variable and can be used to correct for selection bias in the outcome equation.

Both the switching regression models and the instrumental variables approach have their own strengths and limitations. Evaluators who use these techniques should do so with care under the guidance of an econometrician or a statistician.

The regression model (Equation 9.1) also can be utilized to obtain more precise estimates of the magnitude and direction of associations in implementation evaluations. For example, in the evaluation of the high school clinic, the evaluator might be interested in the association between class membership and clinic visits, controlling for other student characteristics. This model can be estimated by omitting the T variable from the model and inserting one or more variables to measure class membership, along with other control variables, such as gender and grade point average.

Regression models also may be used to estimate program effects in the pretest-posttest control group design or the nonequivalent comparison group design. The general form of the model for *comparing the posttest scores of the two groups* is presented below:

$$O = f (T, P, C, I) \tag{9.2}$$

where
- O = Outcome, or posttest score
- T = (0, 1) is a dummy variable
  where 1 = member of treatment group
  and 0 = member of the control group
- P = Pretest score of outcome measure
- C = Control variables
- I = One or more interaction terms

If the regression coefficient for T is statistically significant, the T coefficient is the estimate of the program's effect *on observed outcomes*, controlling for the pretest score of the outcome measure and other factors. In nonequivalent comparison group designs, statistical techniques to correct for potential selection bias also can be applied in Equation 9.2.

If instead the aim of the analysis is to *compare the change in scores between the pretest and posttest* between the two groups, the same model can be used, *inserting the change score as the dependent variable*. If the regression coefficient for T is statistically significant, the T coefficient is the estimate of the program's effect on the *change* in outcomes in the treatment group relative to the control group, controlling for the pretest score of the outcome measure and other factors.

Impact evaluations using single or multiple time series designs with a large number of time points typically employ advanced regression techniques that are beyond the scope of this textbook (McCain and McCleary 1979; McDowall et al. 1980; Ostrom 1978). These types of analyses are best performed with the direction and guidance of a statistician.

Finally, triangulation also is an important method of data analysis in quantitative evaluations of health programs. Health programs are complex entities that are difficult to understand and evaluate. If the goal of the evaluation is to make explicit, specific statements about the causal effects of the program, or what happened in the program during the course of implementation, the evaluator should always have several independent findings giving consistent results before reaching firm conclusions (Luft 1986). Evaluators should explicitly build triangulation into their data analysis plans to make sure that questions are answered based on converging evidence from independent analyses of different sources of data.

SUMMARY

Data collection typically culminates in a "mountain" of information about the program. To avoid being overwhelmed by the data, the evaluation should develop a "question-oriented" data analysis plan that is organized to identify the information required to answer a question, to analyze this information using one or more appropriate techniques, and to formulate an answer to the question(s) based on the results. Qualitative and quantitative analyses can be performed to answer an evaluation question, and confidence in the results can be developed through triangulation.

With the completion of the data analysis, Act II of the evaluation process comes to a close, and the time has come to disseminate results to decision makers and other groups in Act III of the evaluation process, which is the subject of the next chapter.

LIST OF TERMS

Bivariable analysis

Data triangulation

Descriptive analysis

Instrumental variables

Interaction variables

Investigator triangulation

Method triangulation

Multivariable analysis

Switching regression models   Triangulation

Theory triangulation

_____STUDY QUESTIONS

1. How can a question-oriented approach aid the analysis of qualitative information collected in a program evaluation?

2. In quantitative data analysis, how do a program's measures affect the data analysis plan?

3. What are the three types of data analysis? Should multivariable analyses always be performed in quantitative evaluations of program impacts or implementation?

4. What statistical techniques might be used for each impact design described in Chapter 4?

5. What is triangulation in data analysis? What are the four basic types of triangulation? How can triangulation be used in the analysis of qualitative data? In the analysis of quantitative data? In the analysis of both types of data?

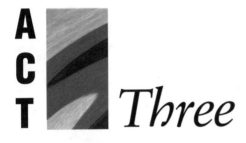

ACT *Three*

USING THE ANSWERS IN DECISION MAKING

CHAPTER 10

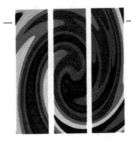

*Disseminating
the Answers to
Evaluation Questions*

After the data are analyzed and each question is answered, Act II comes to a close, but the evaluator still has much work to do. Act III of the evaluation process is opening, and in it the findings and their implications are disseminated to decision makers, interest groups, and other constituents in a political context. A central assumption of Act III is that evaluations are useful only when their results are actually used in some way by decision makers, policymakers, or other groups (Patton 1997; see Chapter 2). To achieve this final milestone, the evaluator sheds the "researcher" role and becomes the "communicator," or the person who informs decision makers about the evaluation's results and recommendations, and who helps them interpret, understand, and apply them in some way.

For the evaluator, however, Act III entails more than simply "delivering the message" to decision makers and interest groups. Just like a play's director brings the story to an end and the audience achieves a "sense of closure" with the play, so must the evaluator achieve closure with decision makers, interest groups, and other participants with whom he or she has worked throughout the evaluation process. In Act III, the evaluator's role is to engage decision makers and other groups, lead them through the act, and bring the play to an end. In this *social process*, the path to closure can be unpredictable, and as the "messenger" delivering the evaluation's results, the evaluator is fully aware that he or she will be the center of attention and may be the target of political attacks when findings and recommended changes oppose the interests of specific groups. Thus, for the evaluator, Act III is all about navigating the social and political terrain in ways that increase the likelihood that findings will actually be used in some way.

In presenting results and recommendations, the evaluator also should decide whether he or she will be an advocate—that is, actively lobbying for change and working with the program to implement recommendations after the evaluation is over (see Chapter 2). In some health organizations, evaluation findings and recommendations without an advocate may go nowhere (Sonnichsen 1994). Action-oriented evaluators who want to be change agents may assume advocacy roles and strive to be influential players in the program's organization.

With these roles in mind, the chapter is organized around the three scenes of Act III. In Scene 1, the answers to the evaluation questions and recommendations are translated from "evaluation language" back into "policy language" so they are understood readily by decision makers. In Scene 2, the evaluator develops a formal plan for disseminating the "policy language" findings to decision makers. Finally, Scene 3 presents methods for increasing the likelihood that evaluation results are actually used by decision makers.

SCENE 1: TRANSLATING ANSWERS BACK INTO POLICY LANGUAGE AND DEVELOPING RECOMMENDATIONS

Translating the Answers

In the Medicare demonstration described in Chapter 3, suppose that the following evaluation question was asked in Act I of the evaluation process:

> What is the effect of the Medicare demonstration on the satisfaction of Medicare enrollees with preventive services?

To answer this question, Medicare enrollees are asked to complete a follow-up survey at the end of the demonstration. The follow-up survey contains a question asking Medicare enrollees in the treatment and control groups to rate their satisfaction on a 0-to-10 scale, where a "0" indicates *extremely dissatisfied* and a "10" indicates *very satisfied*. After the data are collected, a multivariable regression analysis is performed, and based on the results of the statistical analysis, the evaluator answers the question as follows in the technical report:

Controlling for patient characteristics at baseline and the characteristics of the patient's medical office and physician, ordinary least squares regression analysis revealed that the demonstration had a statistically significant and positive effect on enrollee satisfaction with preventive services ($p < .02$). The magnitude of the effect was 2.34, with a 95% confidence interval of 1.84-2.84.

Evaluation has its own, technical language that is understood by evaluators but is viewed as "jargon" at best and "nonsense" at worst by decision makers and those outside the field. If the evaluation findings are presented to decision makers using the above language, decision makers likely will neither hear nor understand the answers to the questions from Act I of the evaluation process. Because the evaluator's goal is to communicate findings in ways that are understood by a variety of audiences, the technical answers must be translated back into policy language (see Chapter 2). For example, the above findings could be presented to a lay audience as follows:

> We found that seniors in the demonstration project were more satisfied with their preventive care than seniors who did not receive the demonstration's services.

In short, for each question asked in Act I, decision makers want to know the "bottom line," and it is the evaluator's job to distill large amounts of data analysis and technical language into a few crisp sentences that can be understood by most people.

Developing Recommendations

In Act I, organizations and decision makers may authorize an evaluation primarily because they are dissatisfied with the status quo and want change. By themselves, the answers to the evaluation questions raised in Act I do not indicate whether or how a program should be changed. As objective, knowledgeable observers of programs, however, evaluators are often well qualified to recommend changes *based on the evaluation's evidence* that may improve a program's processes or outcomes. In some cases, the people authorizing an evaluation in Act I may want only answers to their evaluation questions, without any recommendations. If this is not the case, evaluators may actually lose credibility in Act III if they have no specific changes to recommend (Sonnichsen 1994).

The purpose of recommendations is to convert evaluation findings into "action statements" that identify alternative ways of changing a program (Sonnichsen 1994). To have a realistic chance of being implemented, recommendations (Hendricks 1994; Hendricks and Papagiannis 1990; Sonnichsen 1994) should be

Defensible: Recommendations should be linked to the evaluation findings and be derived directly from the empirical evidence.

Timely: Timeliness is a critical feature—recommendations have little value if they are not ready when decision makers want them, or if decisions have already been made.

Realistic: If implementation of the recommendation appears to be unfeasible, it will likely be ignored by decision makers.

Targeted: Recommendations should indicate who has the authority to approve or disapprove them, and who will be responsible for implementing them, if they are approved.

Simple: Recommendations are more easily understood when they are expressed in clear, simple language.

Specific: Recommendations are more likely to be implemented when they address only one idea and are organized into specific tasks or actions.

The following guidelines are often helpful for developing recommendations (Brandon 1999; Hendricks 1994; Hendricks and Handley 1990; Hendricks and Papagiannis 1990; Sonnichsen 1994).

Invest time: In Act III, the audience may be more interested in the recommendations than in the findings of the evaluation. In many evaluations, however, little time is devoted to developing them, which may dilute their influence.

Start early: Many evaluators do not wait until Act III to begin formulating recommendations. In fact, some evaluators begin in Act I, asking decision makers to propose recommended changes if the evaluation has one set of results, and to propose other recommendations if different results are obtained (Roberts-Gray et al. 1987). Then, when the findings are known, the evaluator is ready to present recommendations already developed by decision makers.

Consider all issues as fair game: When developing recommendations, consider a wide variety of issues and findings in the evaluation, rather than a narrow set of concerns, which may lead to a variety of recommendations. The audience often contains groups with diverse interests, each searching for recommendations that address its own concerns. In a political context, recommendations may be accepted more readily when they offer something for everyone.

Cast a wide net: Good recommendations can come from many different places. Previous evaluations of similar programs may contain recommendations that might apply to the current evaluation. Program staff at all levels are another good source, because their different perspectives often yield good ideas for future steps. Similarly, program clients also are sources to consider in developing recommendations.

Work closely with decision makers and program staff (or, put another way, avoid surprising people): Evaluators may have insufficient expertise to fully understand nuances about the program's history and cultural context, management style and relationships with program staff, and daily operations to compose well-informed recommendations that have good chances of being accepted (Brandon 1999). Recommendations offered solely by evaluators also can be threatening to others. By working closely and honestly with decision makers and program staff, the evaluator can diffuse the threat and work actively to build acceptance of the recommendations. In doing so, however, evaluators may become too involved in their clients' perspectives and lose their independence and objectivity, which may lead to avoidance of controversial issues, equivocation on negative findings, or simply being less candid. Alternatively, the evaluator may favor recommendations that everyone agrees with and ignore recommendations that are controversial but have the potential for major program improvements. Another danger is that a decision maker, intrigued by a preliminary recommendation, may implement it even though the evaluation is incomplete and the recommendation's weaknesses are unknown. Evaluators should anticipate these forms of co-optation and strive to avoid them (see Chapter 2).

Decide whether recommendations should be as general or specific as possible: On one hand, if the specific details of the recommendation are omitted, it may be unclear who should do what, when, and how, and as a result, few or no changes occur. On the other hand, it may be easier to achieve consensus on the ends than on the means of the recommendation. For example, it may be more politically acceptable and less threatening to recommend that "the program's management should be improved" rather than "the program's management should be improved by replacing or re-assigning Person A." By defining only the ends, general recommendations also give program administrators at least some control over how those ends are achieved. General recommendations are not necessarily better than specific ones, or vice versa. For any given program, evaluators must weigh the advantages and disadvantages of being too specific or too general.

Consider program context: Recommendations must have a close "fit" with the program's political, cultural, social, and organizational contexts. Thus, a recommendation that worked well in a previous prenatal care program for Caucasian women may not work in a program targeting Hispanic women. This is another reason to work closely with program staff and clients to verify whether a proposed change will be accepted in a given setting.

Describe expected benefits and costs: A recommendation may have greater appeal when the evaluator describes its expected benefits and the resources required to implement it. A workable advance strategy or plan for implementing a recommendation also may increase its appeal and acceptance. This is an important feature when the evaluator has an up-front commitment to work with the agency to implement the recommendation after the evaluation is completed.

Decide whether change should be incremental vs. fundamental: Evaluation findings may suggest that a program must be changed in fundamental ways (e.g., changing the objectives of the program). Fundamental change, however, is often complex and politically risky. The evaluator should consider whether the goals of the recommendation are more likely to be achieved through fundamental change or a series of incremental improvements that, in the end, lead to the same destination.

Avoid recommending another evaluation: Evaluators can shirk their responsibility in Act III by stating that the results raised more questions than they answered, then recommending another evaluation of the program. Many members of the audience will be dissatisfied with this outcome, and evaluators should avoid falling into this trap by conducting rigorous evaluations, as spelled out in Acts I and II, and by adhering to the ethical principles of evaluation (see Chapter 2).

Different evaluators end their evaluations at different times (Hendricks and Handley 1990). Some evaluators stop after the results are known and presented, others stop after the recommendations are advanced, and still others provide "service after the sale" and help the program implement the recommendations. If the ultimate goal of a recommendation is to improve program performance, then a poorly implemented recommendation does not benefit the program. Evaluators should work with decision makers and program staff to decide whether they should be involved in some way in implementing the recommendations. This decision can be made as early as Act I of the evaluation process, when the scope of the evaluation is determined, or in Act III, when the nature of the recommendations is known.

SCENE 2: DEVELOPING A DISSEMINATION PLAN

Once the findings are translated back into policy language and recommendations are developed, the evaluator's next concern is making sure that everyone is informed about them. One way to increase the likelihood of this outcome is to develop a *dissemination plan*. In the first part of the plan, the evaluator defines all the decision makers, funding agencies, program administrators and clients, and other interest groups who should receive the results and recommendations of the evaluation. This list typically is composed of individuals and groups who played a role in framing the evaluation questions in Act I of the evaluation process, plus other individuals and groups who might be interested in the results.

For each member of the list, the evaluator decides

▶ *What* information to convey

▶ *How* the information should be conveyed

▶ *When* the information should be conveyed

▶ *Where* the communication should be conveyed

▶ *Who* should convey the information

These decisions form the program's dissemination plan. Table 10.1 presents a sample plan for the evaluation of the high school clinic, which was introduced in Chapter 7. In this section, the columns of the table are reviewed.

Target Audience and Type of Information

The first column of the table indicates the target audiences for evaluation results and recommendations. For each audience, the plan indicates (in the second column) what information should be conveyed to its members. Evaluations typically generate much information, and some pieces of the information may be

TABLE 10.1   A Sample Dissemination Plan for an Evaluation of a High School Clinic

Target Audience	Types of Information	Information Formats	Timing of Information	Setting
Clinic director and staff	Progress updates and final results	Oral presentations and brief memos or e-mail messages	Once a month	Meetings with evaluation director and staff
Clinic advisory board	Progress updates	Oral presentations	Quarterly	Board meeting
	Final results and preliminary recommendations	Oral presentations and discussion	Act III	Board meeting
Principal, school administrators, and teachers	Progress updates	Written summary	Quarterly	School mail
	Final results and preliminary recommendations	Oral presentations and discussion	Act III	Group meeting
Officers of Parent Teachers Association (PTA)	Final results and preliminary recommendations	Oral presentation and discussion	Act III	Formal meeting
	Summary of results and recommendations	Parent newsletter	Act III after PTA presentation	Mail
Superintendent of school district and school board	Final results and recommendations	Oral presentation, executive summary, and final report	Act III	Formal meeting

relevant to certain members of the list, whereas other pieces of information are relevant to other members. The evaluator therefore should define explicitly "who should receive what" information in the plan. For example, although the director of the high school clinic may want to read the entire final report, the superintendent of the school district may be interested only in a one-page summary and a chance to discuss the findings with the leaders of the evaluation team.

Format of Information

In the third column, the format of the information should be defined for each audience. In general, there are four modes of conveying results: written, oral, electronic, and visual (Weiss 1998b). In Table 10.1, some information is conveyed orally, such as discussions at regular meetings of the evaluation team, or a formal presentation of final results to the school district's superintendent. Other information is conveyed in a written format, such as through periodic progress updates transmitted by e-mail or documents describing the final results and recommendations of the evaluation. Written communications should be "packaged" in four levels to satisfy the information requirements of different audiences, as described below.

▸ *Comprehensive reports* are for evaluators, researchers, and other audiences who want to know about the details of the evaluation. Table 10.2 lists the content areas often found in final reports of program evaluations (Royse and Thyer 1996; Weiss 1998b; Worthen et al. 1997).

▸ *Ten-page summaries* are excellent for audiences who want to know the facts of the evaluation but do not want to read the full report to discover them. In Table 10.1, for example, summaries might be relevant for teachers and administrators at the high school, as well as members of the advisory board. Staff aides to legislators and other public officials also are receptive to this level of information.

▸ *Two-page executive summaries* are ideal for decision makers who only want to know only the "bottom line" results and recommendations of the evaluation. For a lay audience, a two-page press release that is written in "newspaper language" might be the preferred mode.

▸ In some cases, *250-word summaries* may be essential for decision makers who have only a few minutes to review the evaluation's progress or final results, or to make a decision about program recommendations.

TABLE 10.2   Content Areas of a Final Report for an Evaluation

I. Abstract summarizing main results
II. Executive summary of evaluation results
    A. Brief description of program
    B. Questions asked about the program
    C. Main findings
    D. Recommendations
III. Introduction to the report
    A. Description of the problem that the program addresses
    B. Description of the program's history, activities, beneficiaries, staff, and funding
    C. Description of the program's theory of cause and effect and theory of implementation
IV. Purpose of the evaluation
    A. Description of the questions asked about the program
    B. Description of the answers to these questions found in previous evaluations of similar programs (if any)
V. Methods for answering the evaluation questions
    A. Design of the evaluation
    B. Evaluation setting(s) and population(s)
    C. Selection of study subjects
        1. Source
        2. Sampling method/recruitment
        3. Criteria for eligibility/exclusion of cases
    D. Measures and information
    E. Data collection protocols
        1. Sources (e.g., questionnaire, interview, record review, vital records)
        2. Protocol for typical case
        3. Steps taken to ensure data quality
        4. Statistical power of sample size
    F. Analysis plan and triangulation methods
VI. Results
    A. Characteristics of the sample
    B. Table(s) or figure(s) addressing each research question, progression from univariate, to bivariate, to multivariate analyses; text highlights (but does not duplicate) results shown in tables and figures.
VII. Discussion and conclusions
    A. Interpretation of results
    B. Comparison of results with previous evaluations of similar programs
    C. Confirmation or revision of the program's theory of cause and effect and theory of implementation
    D. Bottom-line conclusions
    E. Evaluation strengths and limitations
VIII. Recommendations
IX. Acknowledgments
X. Appendices
    A. Data collection materials and protocols
    B. Instructions for computing scale scores
    C. Data tables
    D. Transcripts from narrative material

In many evaluations of health programs, the evaluator wants to communicate through written materials with individuals, groups, and institutions that are not directly connected to the program, such as fellow professionals around the country or the world, the general public, or members of Congress. In these cases, the evaluator also can communicate through a wide variety of written materials (Hendricks 1994):

▶ Journal articles and book chapters

▶ Newspaper and magazine articles

▶ Text of speeches or conference proceedings

▶ Brochures

▶ Newsletters

▶ Written testimony

▶ Documents posted on an Internet Web site

Oral presentations and visual aides, such as slides or transparencies, posters, or flip charts, also are common modes of conveying results to decision makers. Oral presentations can be either *informal* or *formal*. As an example of an informal presentation, the evaluator might present progress reports to the high school principal through informal lunch meetings (see Table 10.1). Informal presentations, or "debriefings," also are forums for breaking "bad news"—or negative evidence about the program—to selected audiences (Van Mondfrans 1985; Worthen et al. 1997). Many audiences may have defensive or hostile reactions to negative findings for a variety of reasons, such as fear of being blamed for them, fear that the results will have adverse consequences for the program or themselves personally, a sense of powerlessness or inability to control the situation, or sensitivity toward criticism in any form (for example, see Deyo et al. 1997). This is particularly the case when negative findings are distilled from qualitative evidence, which can reveal the program's problems in vivid detail.

Informal debriefings are useful forums for breaking bad news because the evaluator has more control over *how* an audience hears the message. For example, Worthen et al. (1997) and Van Mondfrans (1985) recommend using "a spoonful of sugar to help the bitter pill go down." That is, the evaluator presents the "good news," or positive findings, about the program first, and then describes the negative results in a straightforward and factual manner but in as positive a perspective as possible. This can be a stand-alone strategy for conveying negative results, or the evaluator may schedule the debriefing after those attending the meeting have reviewed the evaluation's preliminary written report. The latter strategy can be problematic: If the preliminary findings are attacked and prove to be incorrect, the evaluator's credibility may be irreparably damaged, and as a consequence, no one pays much attention to the "final" results when they are disseminated later (Weiss 1998b).

If a debriefing is held, follow-up meetings sometimes are necessary to allow further discussion of negative findings. Some members of the audience may claim the findings are unfair, or they may identify other factors about the program that the evaluator did not consider (Van Mondfrans 1985; Worthen et al. 1997). If the evaluator decides to address these factors and changes are made in the evaluation's final report, the changes should not delete or obscure negative results or allow them to be misinterpreted. When audiences have the opportunity to review negative results, to discuss them with the evaluator, and to offer modifications, those audiences often are more prepared to handle the negative findings when they are released officially.

Evaluators also make formal presentations to a program's audiences. In Table 10.1, for example, the school board may ask the evaluator to make a 5-minute presentation of the evaluation's findings at the next board meeting. In doing so, the evaluator must decide who should present the results to the board members. For example, even though the evaluator may know more than anyone else about the evaluation and its findings, the director of the local health department, who ultimately is accountable for the operation of the high school clinic, might be the "best" person to present the results to the city council and persuade the council to increase the program's budget. On the other hand, if the findings of the evaluation are controversial, elected and appointed officials may be reluctant to be in the "spotlight" of a political controversy. In this case, the responsibility may fall to the evaluator, who should have good presentation skills as well as experience in managing and surviving political conflicts.

Evaluators often use visual aids, such as slides or transparencies, when making oral presentations to audiences. A variety of computer software programs are available for creating visual aids containing text, graphs, and charts. Hendricks (1994) presents guidelines for constructing graphics to illustrate evaluation results. Fink (1993) offers the following guidelines for preparing visual aids and conducting the presentation.

> ▶ The evaluator should do the talking and explaining and let the audience listen. Visuals should be used to focus the audience's attention on the key points of the talk, and the visuals should not distract the audience from listening to the oral presentation.

▶ Each visual should have a title to tell the audience what it is about.

▶ During the talk, the evaluator should describe the program briefly, present the evaluation questions, cover the main methods for answering them, describe results, and then wrap up with conclusions and recommendations.

▶ Tables and figures should be simple to read.

▶ Each slide should be checked for typographical errors.

To illustrate these guidelines, let's suppose that you have been asked to make a 5-minute presentation of the interim results from an evaluation of health clinics in four inner-city junior high schools in New York City (as published by Walter et al. 1996). In 1986, New York School District Six implemented school-based clinics in four public junior high schools in low-income and medically underserved areas of the city. About 81% of the students were Hispanic, mainly children of adult immigrants from the Caribbean, and 10% were African American. Figure 10.1 (pp. 272-280) illustrates how the above guidelines could be applied to develop 10 slides (on average, 2 slides per minute) covering six topics for the presentation (Fink 1993).

Timing of the Information

Next, the evaluator must decide when the information should be presented to each audience. For many programs, it is critical that answers to evaluation questions be presented *before* a decision is made about the program. Thus, if the school board is the relevant audience and a presentation is the best format for conveying the results to the board, the evaluator should find out when the board wants to return to the issues surrounding the program and schedule time on the board's agenda to present the results.

Evaluators also should consider when to release evaluation results. Rather than presenting all findings to everyone at once, partial results can be released to each audience according to a predetermined schedule. As shown in the fourth column of Table 10.1, the clinic director, for example, receives progress reports at least once a month, whereas the clinic advisory board receives them each quarter.

Alternatively, in some evaluations, the answers to some questions are known before the answers to other questions. Rather than waiting until all answers to all questions are known, the evaluation team can release "interim reports" describing the results for questions as each one is answered. By doing so, the

(text continued on p. 281)

Figure 10.1. Example Slides or Overheads for a Short Presentation of Interim Results From an Evaluation of Health Clinics in Junior High Schools

A. Title of the Talk, Affiliation of the Evaluators, and Clinic Sponsors

Evaluation of Health Clinics in Junior High Schools: Interim Results

Prepared by
Name of Evaluator(s)

New York City School District Six
Columbia University of Public Health
Presbyterian Hospital

Slide 1

Figure 10.1. Continued

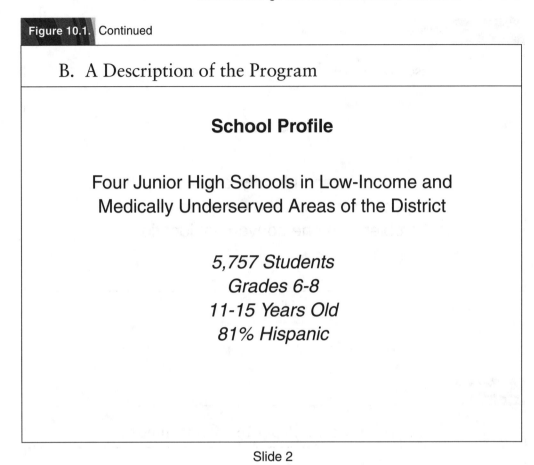

Slide 2

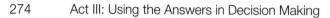
Figure 10.1. Continued

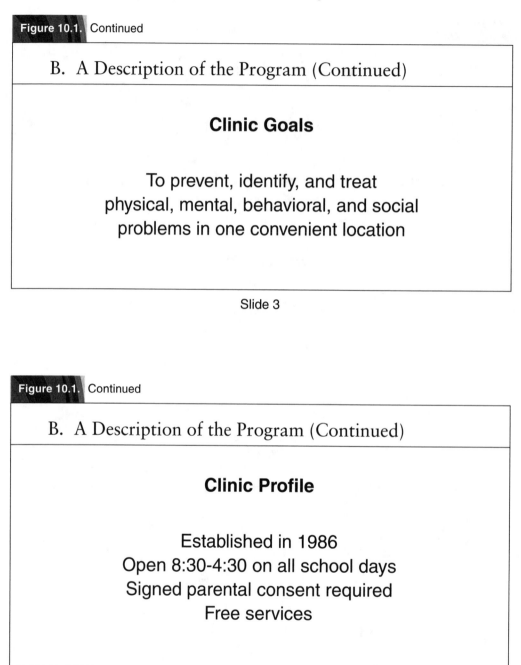

B. A Description of the Program (Continued)

Clinic Goals

To prevent, identify, and treat
physical, mental, behavioral, and social
problems in one convenient location

Slide 3

Figure 10.1. Continued

B. A Description of the Program (Continued)

Clinic Profile

Established in 1986
Open 8:30-4:30 on all school days
Signed parental consent required
Free services

Slide 4

Figure 10.1. Continued

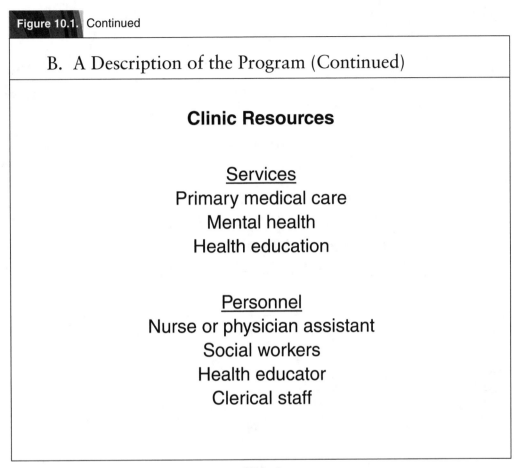

Slide 5

Figure 10.1. Continued

C. The Evaluation Question(s) That the Oral Presentation
Will Answer

Evaluation Question

*Are students who used the
health clinics in the junior high schools
similar to or different from students
who did not use the clinics?*

Slide 6

Figure 10.1. Continued

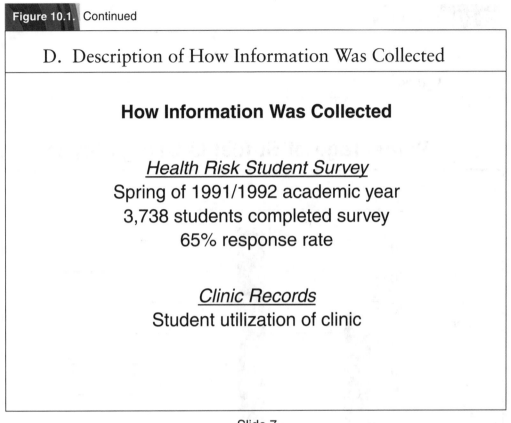

D. Description of How Information Was Collected

How Information Was Collected

Health Risk Student Survey
Spring of 1991/1992 academic year
3,738 students completed survey
65% response rate

Clinic Records
Student utilization of clinic

Slide 7

Figure 10.1. Continued

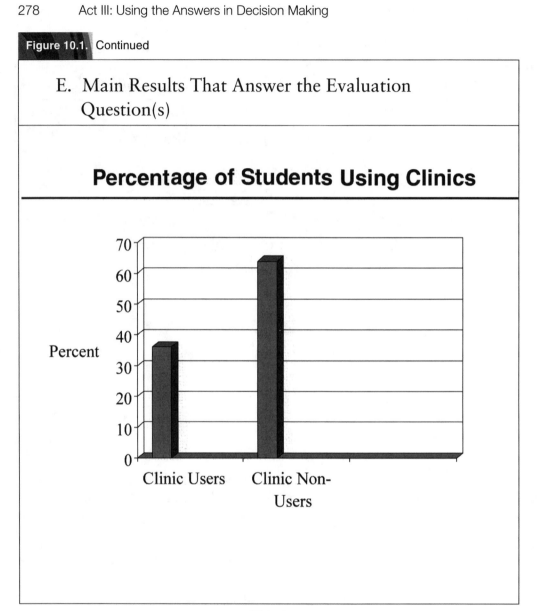

E. Main Results That Answer the Evaluation
   Question(s)

Slide 8

Figure 10.1. Continued

E. Main Results That Answer the Evaluation
   Question(s) (Continued)

	Users (%)	Non-Users (%)
Have sexual intercourse	22*	18
Do not use birth control	22*	13
Have suicide intentions/attempts	16*	12
Have been suspended for fighting	12*	10

* = Statistically significant

Slide 9

Figure 10.1. Continued

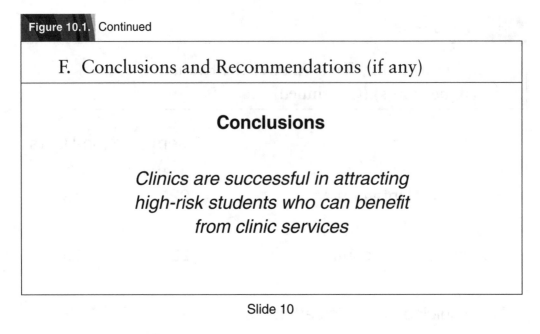

Slide 10

evaluator keeps the audience apprised and involved in the evaluation, builds trust that questions will be answered in an objective and ethical manner, and "sets up" the audience to anticipate and think about recommendations for improving the program.

Similarly, rather than waiting until the end of an evaluation when the "final results" are known, the evaluator can release "preliminary results" and recommendations to audiences early in Act III. As described earlier, preliminary reports are a good way to expose the audiences to sensitive results, tentative conclusions, or recommendations before they are "cast in stone" in the evaluation's final report (Hendricks 1994). In this way, the evaluator can gauge the political and emotional reactions that audiences may have to the information, which can be addressed more fully in the final report. This also can help the evaluator understand, anticipate, and cope with any negative political reactions that may occur when the final results are released.

In addition, although accuracy is prized by evaluators, sometimes errors occur in data collection and analysis that may lead to inaccurate results or conclusions (Worthen et al. 1997). Preliminary reports also provide an opportunity for others to review the early findings and detect errors, which can then be corrected before the final report is released.

Setting

The evaluator also should decide where to present the results to each member of the audience list. In the dissemination plan for the high school clinic evaluation (Table 10.1), the far right column indicates the setting where information will be presented to each audience connected with the program.

For many programs, evaluators also may want to disseminate information to audiences not connected to the program. If the goal is to disseminate results nationally, evaluation results could be presented at professional conferences or through published articles in health journals and bulletins. In contrast, if program advocates want to use the evaluation findings to build support for the program, a public rally may be one of several venues for releasing information and building enthusiasm and support for the program. Clearly, the places for distributing evaluation results will vary depending on the types of audiences on the list and the list's length, what kinds of information they want, the characteristics of the health program, and when the members of the list want the information.

All dissemination plans require time and resources to implement; therefore, after the plan is developed, the evaluator should confirm whether adequate time and sufficient resources exist to carry out the plan. If time and resources fall short, each component of the plan should be reviewed carefully to identify ways of saving time or cutting costs, such as dropping the less central members from the list or choosing more efficient ways of conveying information to members.

SCENE 3: USING THE ANSWERS

How Answers Are Used by Decision Makers

Answers from Act II of the evaluation process are used by decision makers and other groups in different ways. Weiss (1998b) argues that the use of answers by decision makers is a process rather than a single, point-in-time event. Decision makers must first accept the accuracy and relevance of the answers to questions they are facing. Then, the answers interact with what decision makers already know about the program, with their values and beliefs about what is right, with their own interests and the interests of their agencies, with budget and time constraints, and with other factors, to judge the worth of the program and what, if anything, should be done about it. In the end, the answers may or may not be used in one of the following four ways (Weiss 1998a, 1998b).

The first is *conceptual use* of the answers by decision makers, program administrators, and other groups. By answering the questions raised in Act I, evaluations produce new information about what goes on in the program. Conceptual use occurs when this information reveals new insights about the program and this information changes how people think about the program and their understanding of what the program is and how it works. Results from an evaluation may highlight a program's strengths and weaknesses, support or undermine a program's underlying theory of cause and effect and theory of implementation (see Chapter 3), and identify the groups that do and do not benefit from the program. Decision makers may use this information to reorder their priorities, dismiss the problems that led to the program's creation, raise new policy issues, or stimulate others to think in new ways about the program.

The second use is *instrumental*, when answers to the evaluation questions are used by decision makers to change the program, such as expanding the program to other sites, cutting back or terminating the program, or changing how the program is implemented in the field. For health and other types of programs, instrumental use is relatively common *if* any of the following four conditions exist (Weiss 1998a, 1998b):

1. The answers to the questions are not controversial, and people generally agree with the recommended changes (if any);

2. The recommended changes are small, mesh well with the program's operations, and can be implemented easily;

3. The program is relatively stable, and no major changes are planned in the program's leadership, budget, organizational structure and responsibilities, and the types of people served by the program; or

4. The program is facing a crisis or is paralyzed by a problem, and everyone agrees that *something* must be done, but no one knows what to do.

Third, answers to the evaluation questions may be used to *mobilize support* for proposed changes in the program. In some cases, in Act I of the evaluation process decision makers and program administrators may already know what is wrong with the program and how to fix it. *If* the evaluation results support their position, they can use the evaluation findings to legitimize their position, gain the support of interest groups, and implement the recommended changes.

Fourth, answers to evaluation questions may *influence other institutions, decision makers, and interest groups* who are not connected with the program. The audience for evaluation results may extend beyond the decision makers and administrators of a particular program. People in other places may be considering whether to launch the same program or how to change a similar program that is performing badly. To make informed decisions, they may want to know the results of an evaluation of a specific program, as well as the results from different evaluations of the same program implemented in several contexts, which may be available as a meta-analysis (see Chapter 4) or a literature synthesis. This information is useful because it provides evidence about whether previous evaluation findings can be generalized to other places, population groups, and so forth.

When health services are considered, substantial evidence indicates that physicians are slow to adopt improved treatment methods even when there is clear evidence that simple changes in treatment or prevention would promote health and lessen illness and death (Dixon 1990; Lundberg and Wennberg 1997). Thus, just as for health programs, simple dissemination of evidence about the cost-effectiveness of health services does not automatically result in the use of those services by providers. Finding ways to encourage provider adoption of cost-effective treatments is an important area of inquiry in health services research.

In summary, answers to evaluation questions are used in different ways in Act III of the evaluation process. If the answers and their implications are not controversial, they may lead to immediate changes in the program or help program advocates mobilize support for the program. Otherwise, the answers may change people's conceptions of the program, which may have a delayed influence on policy making down the road.

Increasing the Use of Answers in the Evaluation Process

The history of program evaluation indicates that answers to evaluation questions occasionally lead to immediate changes in programs. More often, change is slow and incremental, mainly for two reasons: politics and organizational resistance (Siegel and Tuckel 1985; Weiss 1998b). Some evaluations of health programs are steeped in controversy, with different interest groups holding and promoting conflicting views about what is wrong or right about a program, about the meaning of the answers to the evaluation questions, and what should be done about the program. When Act III becomes politically contentious, change tends to become incremental, if it occurs at all. In this context, the evaluation results may perform an important function by clarifying what decision makers and interest groups are giving up if they fail to support a successful program or settle for a program that is performing poorly.

Changes also may not occur when the organization that is responsible for the program resists implementing them. Many health programs are implemented by organizations; therefore, changing a health program often entails changing the organization that runs the program. Changing an organization, in turn, requires management effort and time, money and other resources, commitment from leadership, and changing the daily routines of staff and how the program and the organization operate. An organization may be reluctant to embrace change until it is convinced that the organization is better off by doing so. Lacking obvious evidence of a better future, an organization may consciously or unconsciously resist change, particularly when change is viewed as a threat to the survival of the organization; too disruptive for staff and the clients served by the program; or offensive to staff, clients, or other groups; or if the organization believes the changes will make things worse by creating new problems or diverting energy away from the problems that the program was created to remedy. In these situations, the "best" that an evaluator often can hope for is incremental change that is acceptable to the organization.

Although evaluators possess some political power in Act III, the power they have is usually too little to overcome the political constraints and organizational resistance surrounding a program. Nevertheless, evaluators can take the following steps to increase the likelihood that answers are actually used in at least one of the four ways described earlier (Chelimsky 1987; Rossi et al. 1999; Shortell and Richardson 1978; Siegel and Tuckel 1985; Solomon and Shortell 1981; Weiss 1998b).

▶ Evaluation findings are more likely to be used if the questions raised in Act I of the evaluation process are actually answered in a clear way, and the answers are communicated directly to decision makers.

▶ Evaluation findings are more likely to be used if decision makers want the results of the evaluation and their policy implications are clear, *and* they receive the information when they want it. This is more likely to happen when decision makers take an active role in framing the evaluation questions in Act I of the evaluation process.

▶ The evaluator can intensify dissemination efforts, relying on more direct rather than passive approaches to inform decision makers.

▶ Evaluation findings confirm the decision makers' general sense of the situation and what must be done about it. Even if the findings are not congruent with the beliefs of decision makers, however, conceptual use of the findings may still occur.

▶ Evaluation findings may stimulate action if they are presented as a "challenge" to the status quo of the agency. Although decision makers tend to favor results that are congruent with their own beliefs, this pattern does not apply to program practices. Decision makers want to know about the program's weaknesses and what can be done to remove them, in either the short or long term.

▶ Evaluators can increase the likelihood that results will be used by conducting rigorous and high-quality evaluations of health programs in Act II of the evaluation process. Decision makers want answers that they are confident are "right" as a defense against interest groups that might attack them when the results are released.

Ethical Issues

In performing the three scenes of Act III, evaluators may encounter serious ethical dilemmas in disseminating evaluation findings. For example, consider the following scenarios:

▶ In Act I, an impact evaluation of a health program is launched because the program director and staff fear that pending budget cuts may lead to a loss of funding and termination of the program. They hire an evaluator from outside the agency to perform the evaluation, hoping the evaluation will produce a "big number" that will provide them with ammunition for defending their beloved program. The impact evaluation, however, reveals that the program had no statistically significant effects. Fearing the evaluation results will do more harm than good, the program director and staff want the evaluator to suppress the findings and not release the report.

▶ An evaluator is hired to perform a fairly "routine" evaluation of the implementation of a new health program. To collect information about the program, the evaluator decides to interview all members of the program's staff. During the course of these informal interviews, the evaluator receives unsolicited information that sexual harassment is occurring regularly in the program, and he or she is uncertain about what to do with this information and whether it should be included in the evaluation's final report (Morris 2000).

▶ The manager of a primary care clinic hires an evaluator to assess the satisfaction of clinic patients. The evaluator decides to use a 10-item patient satisfaction scale that has been used in several previous studies, and he asks 500 adult patients in the waiting room to complete the scale over a 2-week period. Overall satisfaction scores (the average 10-item score for each patient) are very favorable; however, two items on the scale address the clinic's appointment system and amount of time spent in the waiting room, and about 35% of the patients were dissatisfied with these aspects of the clinic. Wanting to make a good impression on the clinic's funding agency, the manager asks the evaluator to report only the favorable overall satisfaction scores.

These and other ethical dilemmas are common in health program evaluation, and dealing with them is one of the most difficult challenges in the evaluation process. The guiding principles for evaluators (American Evaluation Association 1995; see Chapter 2) are general standards for the professional conduct of evaluations of health programs. When tough issues arise, the guiding principles provide an "ethical foundation" that evaluators can use to formulate a position, address the situation, and fulfill their professional responsibilities. When applying the principles to a specific program and ethical issue, there are often several approaches, rather than a single one. One strategy to follow, therefore, is to develop a thorough understanding of the principles and the situation, identify alternative course of action, apply the principles to each course and weigh its advantages and disadvantages, and then choose the course that has the greatest concordance with the guiding principles. Starting in 1999, the *American Journal of Evaluation* has presented cases illustrating how evaluators can perform this exercise successfully.

Evaluating the Evaluation

A central theme of this book is that evaluation is a process composed of distinct elements designed to produce information that is used in some way in decision making. Some evaluations of health programs may be more successful in completing this process than others. When an evaluation is completed, the quality of the evaluation process can be assessed, and this assessment can provide valuable lessons about what went right and what did not in the evaluation, and where improvements could be made. This exercise contributes to the professional growth of the evaluator and is a mechanism for achieving "social closure" among the key participants of the evaluation process.

The Joint Committee on Standards for Educational Evaluation (1994) has developed standards for assessing the quality and fairness of the evaluation process that may be applied to the evaluation of health programs (Centers for Disease Control and Prevention 1999). In total, the Joint Committee presents 30 standards, which are organized into the following four categories:

▶ *Utility standards* require that evaluations produce information that satisfies the information needs of decision makers, funding agencies, interest groups, and other members of the audience.

▶ *Feasibility standards* require that evaluations are feasible—that is, an evaluation can be carried out in the field using a reasonable amount of resources within a given amount of time.

▶ *Proprietary standards* require that evaluations are conducted in an ethical and legal manner, respecting the rights and interests of all participants.

▶ *Accuracy standards* require that evaluations produce sound information and that conclusions and recommendations are linked logically to the data.

The Centers for Disease Control and Prevention (1999) summarizes the standards and describes their application to the evaluation of health programs. The Joint Committee (1994) presents a case study illustrating the application of the standards to an evaluation of an educational program.

SUMMARY

In Act III of the evaluation process, evaluation findings and recommendations are disseminated to decision makers, interest groups, and other constituents. A central assumption is that evaluations have worth only when their results are actually used by decision makers to improve program performance, to formulate new policy, or for other purposes. To encourage use of evaluation findings, evaluators must translate evaluation findings into policy language and formulate recommendations, develop formal dissemination plans to reach all decision makers and interest groups, and take steps that increase the likelihood that results are used in some way. In doing so, evaluators commonly encounter ethical dilemmas, which evaluators can address through the application of the American Evaluation Association's guiding principles for evaluators. Finally, the quality of the evaluation process can be assessed by applying the evaluation standards developed by the Joint Committee on Standards for Educational Evaluation.

LIST OF TERMS

Conceptual use of answers
Dissemination plan
External use of answers by others outside the agency
Instrumental use of answers
Mobilization

STUDY QUESTIONS

1. What is the role of the evaluator in Act III? How is it different from the evaluator's role in the other acts?

2. If you conducted an evaluation of patient and provider satisfaction with the Medicaid program in your state, how would you go about dissemi-

nating your results? Would the nature of your findings affect your dissemination plan? Do political issues affect your plan?

3. What steps can evaluators take to make sure their findings are considered by decision makers, program staff, or other individuals and groups?

CHAPTER 11

Epilogue

All societies have health problems—infectious diseases, injuries, chronic ill-nesses, disabilities, mental distress, and inequitable access to health care, to name but a few. Given the great value that we place on health, large amounts of our society's resources flow to health care organizations to launch health programs and deliver services with the expectation that the problems will be reduced or eliminated. Because uncertainty exists about the causes of many health problems, so does uncertainty exist about the best ways to solve them. Just as mariners rely on gyroscopes to chart a true course, so must health organizations have mechanisms to steer their programs and services in the right direction. Evaluation is one mechanism for doing so. As Cronbach (1982:8) notes, "Social institutions learn from experience; so do clients and political constituencies. The proper function of evaluation is to speed up the learning process by communicating what might otherwise be overlooked or wrongly perceived."

There are at least two ways to speed up this learning process. First, we can draw more from social science theory in the design and evaluation of health programs. That is, to solve a health problem, health professionals try to understand the causes of the problem, develop a program that reduces or eliminates these causes, and then evaluate whether the program worked as intended. For many health problems, causal models can be developed that identify variables having direct and indirect effects on the problem (for example, Chapter 3 presents a simple causal model for low birth weight). Because the elements of causal models are often mediating variables, or the program's mechanisms for producing change, greater use of causal models in health program evaluation might increase our understanding not only of health problems but also of exactly how programs do or do not work to solve them (Grembowski 1984).

Second, we can speed up the learning process by making greater use of meta-analysis. With literally hundreds of programs and services in the field, literally hundreds of evaluations of their performance have accumulated in the literature. A second function of evaluation is to synthesize this evidence to identify the interventions that work, and at what cost, and to understand how the integrity of their implementation affects their success. Although the number of meta-analyses of health services is increasing day by day (Detsky and Redelmeier 1998; Graham et al. 1998; Wright and Weinstein 1998), our knowledge about the performance of health programs is accumulating at a slower pace. For a given health problem, what programs were implemented to solve the problem? What effects did they have on reducing the problem? Did the integrity of program implementation influence these effects? Lipsey illustrates how meta-analysis can define the connection between outcome and implementation for different approaches to solving a health problem (see Table 6.3), and his work should be expanded to also compare costs across programs.

When we blend causal modeling with evidence from meta-analyses, a theory- and evidence-based form of health program evaluation might accumulate over time. Drawing from the discipline of political science, King et al. (1994) articulate how qualitative research can contribute to this effort. When we do this for the major health problems facing society, we can truly "speed up" the accumulation of knowledge about the performance trade-offs of health programs and our perceptions of their worth.

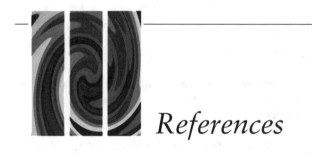

References

Adams PF, Benson V. Current estimates from the National Health Interview Survey, 1989. National Center for Health Statistics. *Vital and Health Statistics* 1990; 10(176).

Aday LA. *Designing and Conducting Health Surveys.* San Francisco: Jossey-Bass; 1996.

Aday LA, Begley C, Lairson DR, Slater C. *Evaluating the Healthcare System: Effectiveness, Efficiency, and Equity.* 2nd ed. Chicago: Health Administration Press; 1998.

Affholter DP. Outcome monitoring. In: Wholey JS, Hatry HP, Newcomer KE, eds. *Handbook of Practical Program Evaluation.* San Francisco: Jossey-Bass; 1994:96-118.

Aiken LS, West SG, Schwalm DE, Carroll JL, Hsiung S. Comparison of a randomized and two quasi-experimental designs in a single outcome evaluation. *Evaluation Review* 1998; 22(2):207-244.

American Evaluation Association, Task Force on Guiding Principles for Evaluators. Guiding principles for evaluators. *New Directions for Program Evaluation* 1995; 66:19-26.

American Psychological Association. *Standards for Educational and Psychological Testing.* Washington, DC: American Psychological Association; 1985.

Andersen RM. Unpublished course syllabus, Evaluation Research: Problems and Techniques in Health Services (Business 589). Chicago: University of Chicago, Graduate School of Business, Center for Health Administration Studies, Graduate Program in Health Administration; 1988 (Autumn).

Anderson OW. *Health Services in the United States: A Growth Enterprise Since 1875.* Ann Arbor, MI: Health Administration Press; 1985.

Astin JA, Harkness E, Ernst E. The efficacy of "distant healing": A systematic review of randomized trials. *Annals of Internal Medicine* 2000; 132(11):903-910.

Bandura A. Self-efficacy mechanism in psychobiologic functioning. In: Schwarzer R, ed. *Self-Efficacy: Thought Control of Action*. Washington, DC: Hemisphere Publishing Company; 1992:355-394.

Banta HD, Luce BR. Assessing the cost-effectiveness of prevention. *Journal of Community Health* 1983; 9(2):145-165.

Baron RM, Kenny DA. The moderator-mediator variable distinction in social psychological research: Conceptual, strategic, and statistical considerations. *Journal of Personality and Social Psychology* 1986; 51(6):1173-1182.

Becker H. Whose side are you on? *Social Problems* 1967; 14:239-248.

Bell JB. Managing evaluation projects step-by-step. In: Wholey JS, Hatry HP, Newcomer KE, eds. *Handbook of Practical Program Evaluation*. San Francisco: Jossey-Bass; 1994:510-533.

Berk RA. An introduction to sample selection bias in sociological data. *American Sociological Review* 1983; 48 (June):386-398.

Berstene TG. Commentary: Process is important. *American Journal of Evaluation* 1999; 20(1):116-118.

Blalock HM. *Causal Inferences in Nonexperimental Research*. New York: W. W. Norton & Company; 1964.

Blalock HM Jr. *Social Statistics*. New York: McGraw-Hill; 1972.

Blumenthal D. The variation phenomenon in 1994. *New England Journal of Medicine* 1994; 331(15):1017-1018.

Borenstein PE, Harvilchuck JD, Rosenthal BH, Santelli JS. Patterns of ICD-9 diagnoses among adolescents using school-based clinics: Diagnostic categories by school level and gender. *Journal of Adolescent Health* 1996; 18(3):203-210.

Boudon R, Bourricaud F. *A Critical Dictionary of Sociology*. Chicago: University of Chicago Press; 1986.

Bourque LB, Clark VA. *Processing Data: The Survey Example*. Sage Series in the Quantitative Applications in the Social Sciences, No. 85. Thousand Oaks, CA: Sage Publications; 1992.

Brandon PR. Involving program stakeholders in reviews of evaluators' recommendations for program revisions. *Evaluation and Program Planning* 1999; 22:363-372.

Brown JB, Adams ME. Patients as reliable reporters of medical care process: Recall of ambulatory encounter events. *Medical Care* 1992; 30(5):400-411.

Brown NL, Penneylegion MT, Hillard P. A process evaluation of condom availability in the Seattle, Washington public schools. *Journal of School Health* 1997; 67(8):336-340.

Buchner D, Casperson C, Carter W, Wagner E, Martin M. *A New Physical Activity Questionnaire for Older Adults*. Unpublished manuscript. Seattle: University of Washington; 1991.

Burt MR. *Practical Methods for Counting the Homeless: A Manual for State and Local Jurisdictions*. Washington, DC: The Urban Institute; 1996.

Campbell DT, Boruch RF. Making the case for randomized assignment to treatments by considering the alternatives. In: Bennett CA, Lumsdaine AA, eds. *Evaluation and Experiment*. New York: Academic Press; 1975:195-297.

Campbell DT, Stanley JC. *Experimental and Quasi-Experimental Designs for Research*. Boston: Houghton Mifflin; 1963.

Carmines EG, Zeller RA. *Reliability and Validity Assessment*. Thousand Oaks, CA: Sage Publications; 1979.

Caudle SL. Using qualitative approaches. In: Wholey JS, Hatry HP, Newcomer KE, eds. *Handbook of Practical Program Evaluation*. San Francisco: Jossey-Bass; 1994:69-95.

Centers for Disease Control and Prevention. Framework for program evaluation in public health. *Morbidity and Mortality Weekly Report* 1999; 48(No. RR-11; September 17).

Charns MP, Schaefer MJ. *Health Care Organizations: A Model for Management*. Englewood Cliffs, NJ: Prentice-Hall; 1983.

Chassin MR, Kosecoff J, Park RE, Winslow CM, Kahn KL, Merrick NJ, Fink A, Keesey J, Solomon DH, Brooks RH. *The Appropriateness of Selected Medical and Surgical Procedures*. Ann Arbor, MI: Health Administration Press; 1989.

Chelimsky E. The politics of program evaluation. *Society* 1987; 25(1):24-32.

Chen HT. *Theory-Driven Evaluations*. Newbury Park, CA: Sage Publications; 1990.

Chen HT, Rossi PH. Evaluating with sense: The theory-driven approach. *Evaluation Review* 1983; 7(3):283-302.

Cherkin DC, Grothaus L, Wagner EH. The effect of office visit copayments on utilization in a health maintenance organization. *Medical Care* 1989; 27(11):1036-1045.

Clancy CM, Eisenberg JM. Outcomes research: Measuring the end results of health care. *Science*. October 9, 1998:245-246.

Cohen J. *Statistical Power Analysis for the Behavioral Sciences*. Rev. ed. New York: Academic Press; 1977.

Cohen J. *Statistical Power Analysis for the Behavioral Sciences*. 2nd ed. Hillsdale, NJ: Lawrence Erlbaum; 1988.

Coile RC. *The Five Stages of Managed Care: Strategies for Providers, HMOs, and Suppliers*. Chicago: Health Administration Press; 1997.

Cole GE. Advancing the development and application of theory-based evaluation in the practice of public health. *American Journal of Evaluation* 1999; 20(3):453-470.

Colton D. The design of evaluations for continuous quality improvement. *Evaluation & the Health Professions* 1997; 20(3):265-285.

Conner RF. Selecting a control group: An analysis of the randomization process in twelve social reform programs. *Evaluation Quarterly* 1977; 1(2):195-244.

Conrad DA, Maynard C, Cheadle A, et al. Primary care physician compensation method in medical care groups: Does it influence the use and cost of health services for enrollees in managed care organizations? *JAMA* 1998; 279(11):853-858.

Cook TD. A quasi-sampling theory of the generalization of causal relationships. *New Directions for Evaluation* 1993; 57(Spring):39-82.

Cook TD, Campbell DT. *Quasi-Experimentation: Design and Analysis Issues for Field Settings*. Boston: Houghton Mifflin; 1979.

Cordray DS, Fischer RL. Synthesizing evaluation findings. In: Wholey JS, Hatry HP, Newcomer KE, eds. *Handbook of Practical Program Evaluation*. San Francisco: Jossey-Bass; 1994:198-231.

Cousins JB, Whitmore E. Framing participatory evaluation. *New Directions for Evaluation* 1998; 80(Winter):5-23.

Cronbach LJ. Coefficient alpha and the internal structure of tests. *Psychometrika* 1951; 16:297-334.

Cronbach LJ. *Designing Evaluations of Educational and Social Programs.* San Francisco: Jossey-Bass; 1982.

Cummings SR, Rubin SM, Oster G. The cost-effectiveness of counseling smokers to quit. *JAMA* 1989; 261(1):75-79.

Curbing Native American smoking [transcript]. "Morning Edition." National Public Radio. December 9, 1998.

Davidoff AJ, Powe NR. The role of perspective in defining economic measures for the evaluation of medical technology. *International Journal of Technology Assessment in Health Care* 1996; 12(1):9-21.

Davis JE. Commentary: Advocacy, care, and power. *American Journal of Evaluation* 1999; 20(1):119-122.

Dean DL. How to use focus groups. In: Wholey JS, Hatry HP, Newcomer KE, eds. *Handbook of Practical Program Evaluation.* San Francisco: Jossey-Bass; 1994:338-349.

Deniston OL, Rosenstock IM. The validity of nonexperimental designs for evaluating health services. *Health Services Reports* 1973; 88(2):153-164.

Dennis ML. Ethical and practical randomized field experiments. In: Wholey JS, Hatry HP, Newcomer KE, eds. *Handbook of Practical Program Evaluation.* San Francisco: Jossey-Bass; 1994:155-197.

Denzin NK. The logic of naturalistic inquiry. In Denzin NK, ed. *Sociological Methods: A Sourcebook.* New York: McGraw-Hill; 1978:6-29.

Detsky AS, Redelmeier DA. Measuring health outcomes—putting gains into perspective. *New England Journal of Medicine* 1998; 339(6):402-404.

DeVellis RF. *Scale Development: Theory and Applications.* Newbury Park, CA: Sage Publications; 1991.

Deyo RA, Diehr P, Patrick DL. Reproducibility and responsiveness of health status measures. *Controlled Clinical Trials* 1991; 12:142S-158S.

Deyo RA, Psaty BM, Simon G, Wagner EH, Omenn GS. The messenger under attack— intimidation of researchers by special-interest groups. *New England Journal of Medicine* 1997; 336(16):1176-1180.

Di Lima SN, Schust CS. *Community Health Education and Promotion: A Guide to Program Design and Evaluation.* Gaithersburg, MD: Aspen; 1997.

Diehr PK, Richardson WC, Shortell SM, LoGerfo JP. Increased access to medical care: The impact on health. *Medical Care* 1979; 27(10):989-999.

Dixon AS. The evolution of clinical policies. *Medical Care* 1990; 28:201-220.

Donabedian A. *Aspects of Medical Care Administration Specifying Requirements for Health Care.* Cambridge, MA: Harvard University Press; 1973.

Doubilet P, Weinstein M, McNeil BJ. Use and misuse of the term "cost-effectiveness" in medicine. *New England Journal of Medicine* 1986; 314:253-256.

Drummond MF, Stoddard GL, Torrance GW. *Methods for Economic Evaluation of Health Programs.* New York: Oxford University Press; 1997.

Duan N, Manning WG Jr., Morris CN, Newhouse JP. A comparison of alternative models for the demand for medical care. *Journal of Business & Economic Studies* 1983; 1(2):115-126.

Durham M, Beresford S, Diehr P, Grembowski D, Hecht J, Patrick D. Participation of higher users in a randomized trial of Medicare reimbursement for preventive services. *The Gerontologist* 1991; 31(5):603-606.

Eastmond N. Commentary: When funders want to compromise your design. *American Journal of Evaluation* 1998; 19(3):392-395.

Edelson JT, Weinstein MC, Tosteson A, Williams L, Lee TH, Goldman L. Long-term cost-effectiveness of various initial monotherapies for mild or moderate hypertension. *JAMA* 1990; 263(3):407-413.

Eisenberg JM. Clinical economics: A guide to the economic analysis of clinical practice. *JAMA* 1989; 262(20):2879-2886.

Elixhauser A, Halpern M, Schmier J, Luce BR. Health care CBA and CEA from 1991 to 1996: An updated bibliography. *Medical Care* 1998; 36(Suppl. 5):MS1-MS9.

Emery DD, Schneiderman LJ. Cost-effectiveness analysis in health care. *Hastings Center Report* 1989; 19(4):8-13.

Faludi A. *Planning Theory.* Oxford, UK. Pergamon Press; 1973.

Fetterman DM. Ethnography. In: Bickman L, Rog DJ, eds. *Handbook of Applied Social Research Methods.* Thousand Oaks, CA: Sage Publications; 1998: 473-504.

Fetterman DM, Kafarian SJ, Wandersman A. *Empowerment Evaluation: Knowledge and Tools for Self-Assessment and Accountability.* Thousand Oaks, CA: Sage Publications; 1996.

Fink A. *Evaluation Fundamentals: Guiding Health Programs, Research, and Policy.* Newbury Park, CA: Sage Publications; 1993.

Fleming GV, Andersen RA. The Municipal Health Services Program: Improving access to primary care without increasing expenditures. *Medical Care* 1986; 24:565-579.

Fleming NS, Becker ER. The impact of the Texas 1989 motorcycle helmet law on total and head-related fatalities, severe injuries, and overall injuries. *Medical Care* 1992; 30(9):832-845.

Floyd RL, Rimer BK, Giovino GA, Mullen PD, Sullivan S. A review of smoking in pregnancy: Effects on pregnancy outcomes and cessation efforts. *Annual Review of Public Health* 1993; 14:379-411.

Friedlander D, Robins P. *Estimating the Effect of Employment and Training Programs: An Assessment of Some Nonexperimental Techniques.* New York: Manpower Demonstration Research Corporation; 1994.

Friedman GD. *Primer of Epidemiology.* New York: McGraw-Hill; 1994.

Fuchs VR. *Who Shall Live? Health, Economics and Social Choice.* New York: Basic Books; 1974.

Fuchs VR. *The Health Economy.* Cambridge: Harvard University Press; 1986.

Garber AM, Weinstein MC, Torrance GW, Kamlet MS. Theoretical foundations of cost-effectiveness analysis. In: Gold MR, Siegel JE, Russell LB, Weinstein MC, eds. *Cost-Effectiveness in Health and Medicine.* New York: Oxford University Press; 1996:25-53.

Gehlbach S. *Interpreting the Medical Literature.* New York: McGraw-Hill; 1993.

Glasgow RE, Vogt TM, Boles SM. Evaluating the public health impact of health promotion interventions: The RE-AIM framework. *American Journal of Public Health* 1999; 89(9):1322-1327.

Gold MR, Patrick DL, Torrance GW, Fryback DG, Hadhorn DC, Kamlet MS, Daniels N, Weinstein MC. Identifying and valuing outcomes. In: Gold MR, Siegel JE, Russell LB, Weinstein MC, eds. *Cost-Effectiveness in Health and Medicine*. New York: Oxford University Press; 1996:82-134.

Gold MR, Siegel JE, Russell LB, Weinstein MC, eds. *Cost-Effectiveness in Health and Medicine*. New York: Oxford University Press, 1996.

Gordon MJ. Research workbook: A guide for initial planning of clinical, social, and behavioral research projects. *Journal of Family Practice* 1978; 7(1):145-160.

Gortmaker SL, Clark CJG, Graven SN, Sobol AM, Deronimus A. Reducing infant mortality in rural America: Evaluation of the Rural Infant Care Program. *Health Services Research* 1987; 22:91-116.

Gottfredson DC, Gottfredson GD, Skroban S. Can prevention work where it is needed most? *Evaluation Review* 1998; 22(3):315-340.

Graham JD, Corso PS, Morris JM, Segui-Gomez M, Weinstein MC. Evaluating the cost-effectiveness of clinical and public health measures. *Annual Review of Public Health* 1998; 19:125-152.

Green LW, Kreuter MW. *Health promotion planning: An educational and ecological approach*. Mountain View, CA: Mayfield Publishing Company; 1999.

Green LW, Lewis FM. *Measurement and Evaluation in Health Education and Health Promotion*. Palo Alto, CA: Mayfield Publishing Company; 1986.

Greene JC. Evaluation as advocacy. *Evaluation Practice* 1997; 18(1):25-35.

Grembowski D. Causal models in plan evaluation. *Socio-Economic Planning Sciences* 1984; 18(4):255-261.

Grembowski D, Blalock AB. Evaluating program implementation. In: Blalock AB, ed. *Evaluating Social Programs at the State and Local Level: The JTPA Evaluation Design Project*. Kalamazoo, MI: W. E. Upjohn Institute for Employment Research; 1990:229-297.

Grembowski D, Cook K, Patrick DL, Roussel AE. Managed care and physician referral. *Medical Care Research and Review* 1998; 55(1):3-31.

Grembowski D, Patrick D, Diehr P, Durham M, Beresford S, Kay E, Hecht J. Self-efficacy and health behavior among older adults. *Journal of Health and Social Behavior* 1993; 34:89-104.

Griffin JF, Hogan JW, Buechner JS, Leddy TM. The effect of a Medicaid managed care program on the adequacy of prenatal care utilization in Rhode Island. *American Journal of Public Health* 1999; 89(4):497-501.

Grossman J, Tierney JP. The fallibility of comparison groups. *Evaluation Review* 1993; 17(5):556-571.

Guyatt G, Walter S, Norman G. Measuring change over time: Assessing the usefulness of evaluative instruments. *Journal of Chronic Disease* 1987; 40(2):171-178.

Haddix AC, Teutsch SM, Shaffer PA. *Decision Analysis and Economic Evaluation*. New York: Oxford University Press; 1996.

Hallam J, Petosa R. A worksite intervention to enhance social cognitive theory constructs to promote exercise adherence. *American Journal of Health Promotion* 1998; 13(1):4-7.

Hannan EL, Kilburn H, Racz M, Shields E, Chassin MR. Improving the outcomes of coronary artery bypass surgery in New York State. *JAMA* 1994; 271(10):761-766.

Hatziandreu EJ, Sacks JJ, Brown R, Taylor WR, Rosenberg ML, Graham JD. The cost effectiveness of three programs to increase use of bicycle helmets among children. *Public Health Reports* 1995; 110(3):251-259.

Hayes R, Baker DW. Methodological problems in comparing English-speaking and Spanish-speaking patients' satisfaction with interpersonal aspects of care. *Medical Care* 1998; 36(2):230-236.

Hedrick SC, Koepsell TD, Inui T. Meta-analysis of home care effects on mortality and nursing home placement. *Medical Care* 1989; 27:1015-1026.

Hendricks M. Making a splash: Reporting evaluation results effectively. In: Wholey JS, Hatry HP, Newcomer KE, eds. *Handbook of Practical Program Evaluation.* San Francisco: Jossey-Bass; 1994:549-575.

Hendricks M, Handley EA. Improving the recommendations from evaluation studies. *Evaluation and Program Planning* 1990; 13:109-117.

Hendricks M, Papagiannis M. Do's and Don'ts for offering effective recommendations. *Evaluation Practice* 1990; 11(2):121-125.

Himmelstein DU, Lewontin JP, Woolhandler S. Who administers? Who cares? Medical administrative and clinical employment in the United States and Canada. *American Journal of Public Health* 1996; 86:172-178.

Hulscher M, Wensing M, Grol R, Van der Weijden T, Van Weel C. Interventions to improve the delivery of preventive services in primary care. *American Journal of Public Health* 1999; 89(5):737-746.

Huntington J, Connell FA. For every dollar spent—the cost-savings argument for prenatal care. *New England Journal of Medicine* 1994; 331(19):1303-1307.

Jaccard J, Turrisi R, Wan CK. *Interaction Effects in Multiple Regression.* Sage Series in the Quantitative Applications in the Social Sciences, No. 72. Thousand Oaks, CA: Sage Publications; 1990.

Joint Committee on Standards for Educational Evaluation. *The Program Evaluation Standards: How to Assess Evaluations of Educational Programs.* Thousand Oaks, CA: Sage Publications; 1994.

Joyce T, Corman H, Grossman M. A cost-effectiveness analysis of strategies to reduce infant mortality. *Medical Care* 1988; 26(4):348-360.

Kane RL, ed. *Understanding Health Outcomes Research.* Gaithersburg, MD: Aspen; 1997.

Kane RL, Henson R, Deniston OL. Program evaluation: Is it worth it? In: Kane RL, ed. *The Challenges of Community Medicine.* New York: Springer; 1974:213-223.

Kaplan A. *The Conduct of Inquiry: Methodology for Behavioral Science.* San Francisco: Chandler Publishing Company; 1964.

Kaplan RM, Bush JW, Berry CC. Health status: Types of validity and the Index of Well-Being. *Health Services Research* 1976; 11:478-507.

King G, Keohane RO, Verba S. *Designing Social Inquiry: Scientific Inference in Qualitative Research.* Princeton, NJ: Princeton University Press; 1994.

King JA, Morris LL, Fitz-Gibbon CT. *How to Assess Program Implementation.* Newbury Park, CA: Sage Publications; 1987.

Kirby D, Brener ND, Brown NL, Peterfreund N, Hillard P, Harrist R. The impact of condom distribution in Seattle schools on sexual behavior and condom use. *American Journal of Public Health* 1999; 89(2):182-187.

Kirk J. *Reliability and Validity in Qualitative Research.* Thousand Oaks, CA: Sage Publications; 1986.

Kish L. *Survey Sampling.* New York: John Wiley and Sons; 1965.

Kolata G. Researchers ask whether prenatal care truly saves money. *New York Times.* November 10, 1994.

Kraemer HC, Thiemann S. *How Many Subjects? Statistical Power Analysis in Research.* Newbury Park, CA: Sage Publications; 1987.

Krieger JW, Connell FA, LoGerfo JP. Medicaid prenatal care: A comparison of use and outcomes in fee-for-service and managed care. *American Journal of Public Health* 1992; 82:185-190.

Kristal AR, Shattuck AL, Henry HJ, Fowler AS. Rapid assessment of dietary intake of fat, fiber, and saturated fat: Validity of an instrument suitable for community intervention research and nutritional surveillance. *American Journal of Health Promotion* 1990; 4:288-295.

Krueger RA. *Focus Groups: A Practical Guide for Applied Research.* Thousand Oaks, CA: Sage Publications; 1994.

Krug EG, Kresnow M, Peddicord JP, Dahlberg LL, Powell KE, Crosby AE, Annest JL. Suicide after natural disasters. *New England Journal of Medicine* 1998; 338(6):373-378.

Landis KR, Koch GG. The measurement of observer agreement for categorical data. *Biometrics* 1977; 33(March):159-174.

Lee PR, Estes CL. *The Nation's Health.* Boston: Jones and Bartlett; 1994.

Leor J, Poole K, Kloner RA. Sudden cardiac death triggered by an earthquake. *New England Journal of Medicine* 1996; 334:413-419.

Levit KR, Lazenby HC, Braden BR, et al. National health expenditures, 1996. *Health Care Financing Review* 1997; 19(1):161-200.

Levit KR, Lazenby HC, Letsch SW, Cowan CA. National health care spending, 1989. *Health Affairs* 1991; 10(1):117-130.

Lima S, Schust CS. *Community Health Education and Promotion: A Guide to Program Design and Evaluation.* Gaithersburg, MD: Aspen; 1997.

Lipscomb J, Weinstein MC, Torrance GW. Time preference. In: Gold MR, Siegel JE, Russell LB, Weinstein MC, eds. *Cost-Effectiveness in Health and Medicine.* New York: Oxford University Press; 1996:214-235.

Lipsey MW. *Design Sensitivity: Statistical Power for Experimental Research.* Newbury Park, CA: Sage Publications; 1990.

Lipsey MW. Juvenile delinquency treatment: A meta-analytic inquiry into the variability of effects. In: Cook TD, Cooper H, Cordray DS, Hartmann H, Hedges LV, Light RJ, Louis TA, Mosteller F, eds. *Meta-Analysis for Explanation: A Casebook.* New York: Russell Sage Foundation; 1992:83-127.

Lipsey MW. Theory as method: Small theories of treatments. *New Directions for Program Evaluation* 1993; 57(Spring):5-38.

Lipsey MW. What can you build with thousands of bricks? Musings on the cumulation of knowledge in program evaluation. *New Directions for Evaluation* 1997; 76(Winter):7-39.

Lipsey MW. Design sensitivity: Statistical power for applied experimental research. In: Bickman L, Rog DJ, eds. *Handbook of Applied Social Research Methods*. Thousand Oaks, CA: Sage Publications; 1998:39-68.

Lipsey MW, Wilson DB. The efficacy of psychological, educational, and behavioral treatment: Confirmation from meta-analysis. *American Psychologist* 1993; 48(12):1181-1209.

Lofland J, Lofland LH. *Analyzing Social Settings: A Guide to Qualitative Observation and Analysis*. Belmont, CA: Wadsworth Publishing; 1984.

Loftin C, McDowall D, Wiersema B, Cottey TJ. Effects of restrictive licensing of handguns on homicide and suicide in the District of Columbia. *New England Journal of Medicine* 1991; 325(23):1615-1620.

Lohr B. *An Historical View of the Research on the Factors Related to the Utilization of Health Services*. Rockville, MD: Bureau for Health Services Research and Evaluation, Social and Economic Analysis Division; January 1972.

Luce BR, Manning WG, Siegel JE, Lipscomb J. Estimating costs in cost-effectiveness analysis. In: Gold MR, Siegel JE, Russell LB, Weinstein MC, eds. *Cost-Effectiveness in Health and Medicine*. New York: Oxford University Press; 1996:176-213.

Luce BR, Simpson K. Methods of cost-effectiveness analysis: Areas of consensus and debate. *Clinical Therapeutics* 1995; 17(1):109-125.

Luepker RV, Perry CL, McKinlay SM, Nader PR, Parcel GS, Stone EJ, Webber LS, Elder JP, Feldman HA, Johnson CC, Kelder SH, Wu M. Outcomes of a field trial to improve children's dietary pattern and physician activity: The Child and Adolescent Trial for Cardiovascular Health (CATCH). *JAMA* 1996; 275:768-776.

Luft HS. Health services research as a scientific process: The metamorphosis of an empirical research project from grant proposal to final report. *Health Services Research* 1986; 21:563-584.

Lundberg GD, Wennberg JE. *JAMA* theme issue on quality of care: A new proposal and call to action. *JAMA* 1997; 278:1615-1616.

MacMahon B, Trichopoulus D. *Epidemiology: Principles and Methods*. Boston: Little, Brown and Company; 1996.

Maddala GS. *Limited-Dependent and Qualitative Variables in Econometrics*. Cambridge, UK: Cambridge University Press; 1983.

Marcantonio RJ, Cook TD. Convincing quasi-experiments: The interrupted time series and regression-discontinuity designs. In: Wholey JS, Hatry HP, Newcomer KE, eds. *Handbook of Practical Program Evaluation*. San Francisco: Jossey-Bass; 1994:133-154.

Mark DB, Hlatky MA, Califf RM, et al. Cost effectiveness of thrombolytic therapy with tissue plasminogen activator as compared with streptokinase for acute myocardial infarction. *New England Journal of Medicine* 1995; 332:1418-1424.

Mark MM, Shotland RL. *Multiple Methods in Program Evaluation*. New Directions for Program Evaluation, No. 35. San Francisco: Jossey-Bass; 1987.

Marmor TR. Forecasting American health care: How we got here and where we might be going. *Journal of Health Politics, Policy, and Law* 1998; 23(3):551-571.

Martin D, Diehr P, Price KF, Richardson WC. Effect of a gatekeeper plan on health services use and charges: A randomized trial. *American Journal of Public Health* 1989; 79:1628-1632.

Masters BA. Bid to help women saving men's lives; Study: Domestic-violence programs keep batterers alive. *Seattle Times* (from the *Washington Post*), March 15, 1999:A1.

Maxwell JA. Designing a qualitative study. In: Bickman L, Rog DJ, eds. *Handbook of Applied Social Research Methods*. Thousand Oaks, CA: Sage Publications; 1998:69-100.

McCain LJ, McCleary R. The statistical analysis of the simple interrupted time-series quasi-experiment. In: Cook TD, Campbell DT, eds. *Quasi-Experimentation: Design and Analysis Issues for Field Settings*. Boston: Houghton Mifflin; 1979:233-293.

McDowall D, McCleary R, Meidinger EE, Hay RA. *Interrupted Time Series Analysis*. Sage Series in the Quantitative Applications in the Social Sciences, No. 21. Thousand Oaks, CA: Sage Publications; 1980.

McDowell CL. Standardized tests and program evaluation: Inappropriate measures in critical times. *New Directions for Program Evaluation* 1992; 53:45-54.

McGinnis JM, Foege WH. Actual causes of death in the United States. *JAMA* 1993; 270(18):2207-2212.

McGraw SA, Sellers DE, Stone EJ, Bebchuk J, Edmundson EW, Johnson CC, Bachman KJ, Luepker RV. Using process data to explain outcomes: An illustration from the Child and Adolescent Trial for Cardiovascular Health (CATCH). *Evaluation Review* 1996; 20(3):291-312.

Meischke H, Finnegan J, Eisenberg M. What can you teach about cardiopulmonary resuscitation (CPR) in 30 seconds? *Evaluation and the Health Professions* 1999; 22(1):44-59.

Mellor S, Mark MM. A quasi-experimental design for studies on the impact of administrative decisions: Applications and extensions of the regression-discontinuity design. *Organizational Research Methods* 1998; 1(3):315-333.

Merriam SB. *Qualitative Research and Case Study Applications in Education*. San Francisco: Jossey-Bass; 1998.

Miles MB, Huberman AM. *Qualitative Data Analysis: A Sourcebook of New Methods*. Thousand Oaks, CA: Sage Publications; 1984.

Miles MB, Huberman AM. *Qualitative Data Analysis: An Expanded Sourcebook*. Thousand Oaks, CA: Sage Publications; 1994.

Miller DC. *Handbook of Research Design and Social Measurement*. Newbury Park, CA: Sage Publications; 1991.

Mintzberg H. *Structure in Fives: Designing Effective Organizations*. Englewood Cliffs, NJ: Prentice-Hall; 1983.

Mohr LB. *Impact Analysis for Program Evaluation*. Chicago: The Dorsey Press; 1988.

Mohr LB. *Impact Analysis for Program Evaluation*. Thousand Oaks, CA: Sage Publications; 1995.

Morris LL, Fitz-Gibbon CT. *How to Measure Program Implementation*. Thousand Oaks, CA: Sage Publications; 1978.

Morris M. Ethical challenges. *American Journal of Evaluation* 1998; 19(3):381-384.

Morris M. The case of the desperate staff. *American Journal of Evaluation* 1999; 20(1):115.

Morris M. The off-the-record case. *American Journal of Evaluation* 2000; 21(1):121.

Moskowitz DB. Looking for new ways to measure the payoff from employer health benefits. *Perspectives on the Marketplace* (suppl. to *Medicine and Health*). May 4, 1998:1-2.

Namboodiri NK, Carter LF, Blalock HM. *Applied Multivariate Analysis and Experimental Design*. New York: McGraw-Hill; 1975.

Neuhauser D, Yin XP. Deciding whether a new test/measure is useful. *Medical Care* 1991; 29(8):685-689.

Newhouse JP. Controlled experimentation as research policy. In: Ginzberg E, ed. *Health Services Research: Key to Health Policy*. Cambridge, MA: Harvard University Press; 1991:161-194.

Newhouse JP, McClellan M. Econometrics in outcomes research: The use of instrumental variables. *Annual Review of Public Health* 1998; 19:17-34.

Nunnally JC. *Educational Measurement and Evaluation*. New York: McGraw-Hill; 1972.

Orwin RG, Sonnefeld LJ, Cordray DS, Pion GM, Perl HI. Constructing quantitative implementation scales from categorical services data: Examples from a multisite evaluation. *Evaluation Review* 1998; 22(2):245-288.

Ostrom CW. *Time Series Analysis: Regression Techniques*. Sage Series in the Quantitative Applications in the Social Sciences, No. 9. Thousand Oaks, CA: Sage Publications; 1978.

O'Sullivan E, Burleson GW, Lamb WE. Avoiding evaluation cooptation: Lessons from a renal dialysis evaluation. *Evaluation and Program Planning* 1985; 8(3):255-259.

Palumbo DJ, ed. *The Politics of Program Evaluation*. Newbury Park, CA: Sage Publications; 1987.

Pardes H, Manton KG, Lander ES, Tolley HD, Ullian AD, Palmer H. Effects of medical research on health care and the economy. *Science*. January 1, 1999:36-37.

Patrick DL, Beresford SA, Ehreth J, Diehr P, Picciano J, Durham M, Grembowski D. Interpreting excess mortality in a prevention trial of older adults. *International Journal of Epidemiology* 1995; 24(Suppl. 1 Pt. 3):S27-S33.

Patrick DL, Erickson P. *Health Status and Health Policy: Quality of Life in Health Care Evaluation and Resource Allocation*. New York: Oxford University Press; 1993.

Patrick DL, Grembowski D, Durham ML, Beresford SA, Diehr P, Ehreth J, Hecht J, Picciano J, Beery W. Cost and outcomes of Medicare reimbursement for HMO preventive services. *Health Care Financing Review* 1999; 20(4):25-43.

Patton MQ. *How to Use Qualitative Methods in Evaluation*. Thousand Oaks, CA: Sage Publications; 1987.

Patton MQ. *Qualitative Evaluation and Research Methods*. Thousand Oaks, CA: Sage Publications; 1990.

Patton MQ. *Utilization-Focused Evaluation: The New Century Text*. Thousand Oaks, CA: Sage Publications; 1997.

Pentz MA, Trebow EA, Hansen WB, MacKinnon DP, Dwyer JH, Johnson CA, Flay BR, Daniels S, Cormack C. Effects of program implementation on adolescent drug use behavior: The Midwestern Prevention Project (MPP). *Evaluation Review* 1990; 14(3):264-289.

Petitti DB. *Meta-Analysis, Decision Analysis, and Cost-Effectiveness Analysis*. New York: Oxford University Press; 1994.

Phillips KA, Holtgrave DR. Using cost-effectiveness/cost-benefit analysis to allocate health resources: A level playing field for prevention? *American Journal of Preventive Medicine* 1997; 13(1):18-25.

Pierce JP, Gilpin EA, Emery SL, White MM, Rosbrook B, Berry CC. Has the California tobacco control program reduced smoking? *JAMA* 1998; 280(10):893-899.

President and Fellows of Harvard College. *Lead Poisoning, Parts A and B* (Case Program, John F. Kennedy School of Government, Documents C14-75-123.0 and C14-75-124.0). Cambridge, MA: Harvard University; 1975.

Pressman JL, Wildavsky A. *Implementation*. Berkeley: University of California Press; 1984.

Radloff LS. The CES-D scale: A self-report depression scale for research in the general population. *Applied Psychological Measurement* 1977; 1:385-401.

Reichardt CS. Estimating the effects of community prevention trials: Alternative designs and methods. In: Holder HD, Howard JM, eds. *Community Prevention Trials for Alcohol Problems: Methodological Issues*. Westport, CT: Praeger; 1992:137-158.

Reichardt CS, Cook TS. Beyond qualitative versus quantitative methods. In: Cook TS, Reichardt CS, eds. *Qualitative and Quantitative Methods in Evaluation Research*. Thousand Oaks, CA: Sage Publications; 1979:7-32.

Reichardt CS, Mark MM. Quasi-experimentation. In: Bickman L, Rog DJ, eds. *Handbook of Applied Social Research Methods*. Thousand Oaks, CA: Sage Publications; 1998:193-228.

Reid RJ. A cost-benefit analysis of syringe exchange programs. *Journal of Health & Social Policy* 2000; 11(4):41-57.

Relman AS. Assessment and accountability: The third revolution in medical care. *New England Journal of Medicine* 1988; 319:1220-1222.

Reynolds AJ. Confirmatory program evaluation: A method for strengthening causal inference. *American Journal of Evaluation* 1998; 19(2):203-221.

Roberts-Gray C, Buller A, Sparkman A. Linking data with action: Procedures for developing recommendations. *Evaluation Review* 1987; 11:678-684.

Rog, DJ. Constructing natural "experiments." In: Wholey JS, Hatry HP, Newcomer KE, eds. *Handbook of Practical Program Evaluation*. San Francisco: Jossey-Bass; 1994:119-132.

Rogers LW, Bergman AB, Rivara FP. Promoting bicycle helmets to children: A campaign that worked. *Journal of Musculoskeletal Medicine* 1991; 8:64-77.

Rossi PH. Advances in quantitative evaluation, 1987-1996. *New Directions for Evaluation* 1997; 76(Winter):57-68.

Rossi PH, Freeman HE. *Evaluation: A Systematic Approach*. Newbury Park, CA: Sage Publications; 1993.

Rossi PH, Freeman HE, Lipsey MW. *Evaluation: A Systematic Approach*. Thousand Oaks, CA: Sage Publications; 1999.

Royse D, Thyer BA. *Program Evaluation: An Introduction*. Chicago: Nelson-Hall; 1996.

Russell LB. The role of prevention in health reform. *New England Journal of Medicine* 1993; 329(5):252-254.

Russell LB, Siegel JE, Daniels N, Gold MR, Luce BR, Mandelblatt JS. Cost-effectiveness analysis as a guide to resource allocation in health: Roles and limitations. In: Gold MR, Siegel JE, Russell LB, Weinstein MC, eds. *Cost-Effectiveness in Health and Medicine.* New York: Oxford University Press; 1996:3-24.

St. Pierre RG. *Management and Organizations for Program Evaluation.* New Directions for Program Evaluation, No. 18. San Francisco: Jossey-Bass; 1983.

Salant P, Dillman DA. *How to Conduct Your Own Survey.* New York: John Wiley and Sons; 1994.

Scheirer MA. *Program Implementation.* Thousand Oaks, CA: Sage Publications; 1981.

Scheirer MA. Designing and using process evaluation. In: Wholey JS, Hatry HP, Newcomer KE, eds. *Handbook of Practical Program Evaluation.* San Francisco: Jossey-Bass; 1994:40-68.

Scheirer MA. Commentary: Evaluation planning is the heart of the matter. *American Journal of Evaluation* 1998; 19(3):385-391.

Scheirer MA, Shediac MC, Cassady CE. Measuring the implementation of health promotion programs: The case of the Breast and Cervical Cancer Program in Maryland. *Health Education Research* 1995; 10(1):11-25.

Schlesinger M. On the limits of expanding health care reform: Chronic care in prepaid settings. *The Milbank Quarterly* 1986; 64(2):189-215.

Schlesinger M, Gray B. A broader vision for managed care, part 1: Measuring the benefit to communities. *Health Affairs* 1998; 17(3):152-168.

Schnelle JF, Kirchner RE, Macrae JW, McNess MP, Eck RH, Snodgrass S, Casey JD, Uselton PH Jr. Police evaluation research: An experimental and cost-benefit analysis of a helicopter patrol in a high-crime area. *Journal of Applied Behavior Analysis* 1978; 11:11-21.

Schulman KA, Berlin JA, Harless W, Kerner JF, Sistrun S, Gersh BJ, Dube R, Taleghani CK, Burke JE, Williams S, Eisenberg JM, Escarce JJ. The effect of race and sex on physicians' recommendations for cardiac catheterization. *New England Journal of Medicine* 1999; 340(8):618-626.

Schweitzer SO, Atchison KA, Lubben JE, Mayer-Oakes SA, De Jong FJ, Matthias RE. Health promotion and disease prevention for older adults: Opportunity for change or preaching to the converted? *American Journal of Preventive Medicine* 1994; 10(4):223-229.

Shadish WR Jr., Cook TD, Leviton LC. *Foundations of Program Evaluation.* Newbury Park, CA: Sage Publications; 1991.

Sheehan TJ. Stress and low birth weight: A structural modeling approach using real life stressors. *Social Science and Medicine* 1998; 47(10):1503-1512.

Shortell SM. Suggestions for improving the study of health program implementation. *Health Services Research* 1984; 19(1):117-125.

Shortell SM. The emergence of qualitative methods in health services research. *Health Services Research* 1999; 34(Suppl., Pt. 2):1083-1090.

Shortell SM, Kaluzny AD. *Health Care Management: Organization Design and Behavior.* Albany, NY: Delmar Thompson Learning; 2000.

Shortell SM, McNerney WJ. Criteria and guidelines for reforming the U.S. health care system. *New England Journal of Medicine* 1990; 322(7):463-467.

Shortell SM, Richardson WC. *Health Program Evaluation.* St. Louis, MO: C. V. Mosby Company; 1978.

Shrout PE, Yager TJ. Reliability and validity of screening scales: Effect of reducing scale length. *Journal of Clinical Epidemiology* 1989; 42(1):69-78.

Siegel JE, Weinstein MC, Russell LB, Gold MR. Recommendations for reporting cost-effectiveness analyses. *JAMA* 1996; 276(16):1339-1341.

Siegel JE, Weinstein MC, Torrance GW. Reporting cost-effectiveness studies and results. In: Gold MR, Siegel JE, Russell LB, Weinstein MC, eds. *Cost-Effectiveness in Health and Medicine.* New York: Oxford University Press; 1996:276-303.

Siegel KL, Tuckel P. The utilization of evaluation research: A case analysis. *Evaluation Review* 1985; 9(3):307-328.

Silverman M, Ricci EM, Gunter MJ. Strategies for increasing the rigor of qualitative methods in evaluations of health care programs. *Evaluation Review* 1990; 14(1):57-74.

Simon JL. *Basic Research Methods in Social Science: The Art of Empirical Investigation.* New York: Random House; 1969.

Sisk JE. The cost of prevention: Don't expect a free lunch. *JAMA* 1993; 269(13):1710, 1715.

Sisk JE, Gorman SA, Reisinger AL, Glied SA, DuMouchel WH, Hynes MM. Evaluation of Medicaid managed care: Satisfaction, access, and use. *JAMA* 1996; 276:50-55.

Snedecor GW, Cochran WG. *Statistical Methods.* Ames: Iowa State University Press; 1980.

Solomon MA, Shortell SM. Designing health policy research for utilization. *Health Policy Quarterly* 1981; 1(3):216-237.

Sonnichsen RC. Evaluators as change agents. In: Wholey JS, Hatry HP, Newcomer KE, eds. *Handbook of Practical Program Evaluation.* San Francisco: Jossey-Bass; 1994:534-548.

Srinivasan S, Levitt L, Lundy J. Wall Street's love affair with health care. *Health Affairs* 1998; 17(4):126-131.

Stewart DW, Shamdasani PN. Focus group research: Exploration and discovery. In: Bickman L, Rog DJ, eds. *Handbook of Applied Social Research Methods.* Thousand Oaks, CA: Sage Publications; 1998:505-526.

Stouthamer-Loeber M, van Kammen WB. *Data Collection and Management: A Practical Guide.* Thousand Oaks, CA: Sage; 1995.

Suchman EA. *Evaluative Research: Principles and Practice in Public Service & Social Action Programs.* New York: Russell Sage Foundation; 1967.

Sudman S, Bradburn NM. *Asking Questions: A Practical Guide to Questionnaire Design.* San Francisco: Jossey-Bass; 1982.

Tengs TO, Adams ME, Pliskin JS, Safran DG, Siegel JE, Weinstein MC, Graham JD. Five-hundred life-saving interventions and their cost-effectiveness. *Risk Analysis* 1995; 15(3):369-390.

Tesch R. *Qualitative Research: Analysis Types and Software Tools.* London: Falmer Press; 1990.

Torrance GW, Siegel JE, Luce BR. Framing and designing the cost-effectiveness analysis. In: Gold MR, Siegel JE, Russell LB, Weinstein MC, eds. *Cost-Effectiveness in Health and Medicine*. New York: Oxford University Press; 1996:54-81.

Trochim W. The regression-discontinuity design. In: Sechrest L, Perrin E, Bunker J, eds. *Research Methodology: Strengthening Causal Interpretations of Nonexperimental Data* (DHHS Publication No. (PHS) 90-3454). Rockville, MD: Agency for Health Care Policy and Research; May 1990:119-139.

Udvarhelyi IS, Jennison K, Phillips RS, Epstein AM. Comparison of the quality of ambulatory care for fee-for-service and prepaid plans. *Annals of Internal Medicine* 1991; 115(5):394-400.

Unutzer J, Patrick DL, Simon G, Grembowski D, Walker E, Rutter C, Katon W. Depressive symptoms and the cost of health services in HMO patients aged 65 years and older: A 4-year prospective study. *JAMA* 1997; 277(20):1618-1623.

Urban N. *Cost-Effectiveness Analysis*. Class presentation in course HSERV 522, Health Program Evaluation, University of Washington, January 25, 1998.

U.S. Department of Health and Human Services (DHHS). *Healthy People 2000* (DHHS Publication No. (PHS) 91-50212). Washington, DC: Superintendent of Documents, Government Printing Office; 1991.

Van Mondfrans A. *Guidelines for Reporting Evaluation Findings*. Unpublished manuscript. Provo, UT: Brigham Young University; 1985.

Veney JE, Kaluzny AD. *Evaluation and Decision Making for Health Services*. Chicago: Health Administration Press; 1998.

Wagenaar AC. Effects of the raised legal drinking age on motor vehicle accidents in Michigan. *HSRI Research Review* 1981; 11(4):1-8.

Wagenaar AC. Preventing highway crashes by raising the legal minimum age for drinking: The Michigan experience 6 years later. *Journal of Safety Research* 1986; 17:101-109.

Walter HJ, Vaughan RD, Armstrong B, Krakoff RY, Tiezzi L, McCarthy JF. Characteristics of users and nonusers of health clinics in inner-city junior high schools. *Journal of Adolescent Health* 1996; 18(5):344-348.

Ware JE Jr., Bayliss MS, Rogers WH, Kosinski M, Tarlov AR. Differences in 4-year health outcomes for elderly and poor, chronically ill patients treated in HMO and fee-for-service systems. *JAMA* 1996; 276(13):1039-1047.

Warner KE. Issues in cost effectiveness in health care. *Journal of Public Health Dentistry* 1989; 49(5):272-278.

Warner KE, Luce BR. *Cost-Benefit and Cost-Effectiveness Analysis in Health Care: Principles, Practice and Potential*. Ann Arbor, MI: Health Administration Press; 1982.

Webb EJ, Campbell DT, Schwartz RD, Sechrest L. *Unobtrusive Measures: Nonreactive Research in the Social Sciences*. Chicago: Rand McNally College Publishing Company; 1966.

Weinstein MC, Stason WB. Foundations of cost-effectiveness analysis for health and medical practices. *New England Journal of Medicine* 1977; 296(13):716-721.

Weiss CH. *Evaluation Research*. Englewood Cliffs, NJ: Prentice-Hall; 1972.

Weiss CH. Ideology, interests, and information: The basis of policy positions. In: Callahan D, Jennings B, eds. *Ethics, the Social Sciences, and Policy Analysis*. New York: Plenum Press; 1983:213-245.

Weiss CH. Nothing as practical as a good theory: Exploring the theory-based evaluation for comprehensive community initiative for children and families. In: Connel JP, Kubisch AC, Schorr LB, Weiss CH, eds. *New Approaches to Evaluating Community Initiatives: Concepts, Methods, and Contexts*. Washington, DC: The Aspen Institute; 1995:65-92.

Weiss CH. Theory-based evaluation: Past, present, and future. *New Directions for Evaluation* 1997; 76(Winter):41-55.

Weiss CH. *Evaluation: Methods for Studying Programs and Policies*. Upper Saddle River, NJ: Prentice Hall; 1998a.

Weiss CH. Have we learned anything new about the use of evaluation? *American Journal of Evaluation* 1998b; 19(1):21-33.

Wilder CS. *Physician Visits, Volume, and Interval Since Last Visit, U.S., 1969* (Series 10, No. 75, DHEW Publication No. (HSM) 72-1064). Rockville, MD: National Center for Health Statistics; July 1972.

Wilson DB. *The Role of Method in Treatment Effect Estimates: Evidence From Psychological, Behavioral, and Educational Meta-Analyses* [dissertation]. Claremont, CA: Claremont Graduate School; 1995.

Windsor RA, Cutter G, Morris J, Reese Y, Manzella B, Bartlett EE, Samuelson C, Spanos D. Effectiveness of self-help smoking cessation interventions for pregnant women in public health maternity clinics: A randomized trial. *American Journal of Public Health* 1985; 75(12):1389-1392.

Windsor RA, Warner KE, Cutter GR. A cost-effectiveness analysis of self-help smoking cessation methods for pregnant women. *Public Health Reports* 1988; 103(1):83-88.

Worthen BR, Sanders JR, Fitzpatrick JL. *Program Evaluation: Alternative Approaches and Practical Guidelines*. New York: Longman; 1997.

Wright JC, Weinstein MC. Gains in life expectancy from medical interventions—standardizing data or outcomes. *New England Journal of Medicine* 1998; 339(6):380-386.

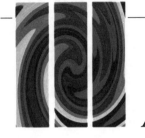

Author Index

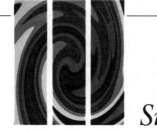

Subject Index

About the Author

David Grembowski, Ph.D., is a professor in the Department of Health Services, School of Public Health and Community Medicine, and the Department of Dental Public Health Sciences, School of Dentistry, at the University of Washington. He has taught health program evaluation to graduate students for more than 10 years. His evaluation interests are the performance of health programs and health care systems. He is conducting an evaluation of managed care and its influence on physician referrals and outcomes of care. He is also directing an evaluation examining associations between managed care, the patient-physician relationship, and health outcomes. His prevention studies have addressed the cost-effectiveness of preventive services for older adults, the effects of fluoridation on oral health and dental expenditures, and the effects of financial incentives on dentist adoption of preventive technologies. Other work includes the evaluation of a partnership program to boost access to dental care among Medicaid-covered preschool children and studies estimating the impact of insurance on the demand for dental care.